Wake the Health Up!

...YOUR LiFE DEPENDS ON iT!

DEVRA BETTS

Each person's physical, emotional, and spiritual condition is unique. The instruction in this book isn't intended to replace or interrupt the reader's one-on-one relationship with a physician or other healthcare professional. Please consult your doctor for matters pertaining to your specific health, exercise, and diet. The information contained within these pages in not intended as medical advice.

Copyright Page – Wake the Health Up © 2018 by Devra Betts

All rights reserved. No part of this publication may be reproduced, distributed, or transmitted in any form or by any means, including photocopying, recording, or other electronic or mechanical methods, including information storage and retrieval systems, without the prior written permission of the publisher or author, except in the case of brief quotations embodied in critical reviews and certain other noncommercial uses permitted by copyright law. For permission requests, email the author at devra@devrabetts.com.

To contact the author, visit devrabetts.com
ISBN 9781730713729
Printed in the United States of America

TABLE OF CONTENTS

FOREWORD	i
...A NOTE FROM THE AUTHOR	1
INTRODUCTION	3
MY JOURNEY	9
WHAT DO *YOU* WANT?	21
YOUR JOURNEY BEGINS HERE	25
MINDSET—WHERE CHANGE BEGINS	33
THE ROOT OF IT!	37
IT'S GENETIC! IS IT THAT SIMPLE?	45
A TOOLKIT FOR OPTIMAL HEALTH ~ MIND, BODY, & SPIRIT	47
THERE'S TOO MUCH ON MY PLATE!	49
HAND OVER THE DONUT AND NO ONE GETS HURT!	53
GET OFF THE DIET ROLLER COASTER	59
WHAT'S FOOD GOT TO DO WITH IT?	65
ON THE INSIDE TRACT	69
CLEAN IT UP, CLEAR IT OUT.	81
HONEY, WE HAVE COMPANY!	89

ABOUT ANTiBiOTiCS...	95
MOVE iT, MOVE iT, MOVE iT!	101
GET YOUR Z'S THE BODY iS UP TO SOMETHiNG GOOD!	107
EAT CLEAN?	115
LET'S GET COOKiNG!	
YOUR KiTCHEN—THE HEART OF THE HOME.	123
GO GREEN! RED, PURPLE, ORANGE AND YELLOW TOO!	137
A GRAiN OF SALT WiTH A SiDE OF iODiNE	143
GiMME COFFEE!	147
WHAT'S iN A LABEL?	155
SPEAKiNG OF SUGAR	165
OBESiTY...iT'S AN EPiDEMiC!	170
THE AiR WE BREATHE	175
TiDY UP!	183
HEART OF FORGiVENESS	187
TOO BLESSED TO BE STRESSED!	191
GiVE YOURSELF SOME LOVE	195
SUPPLEMENTS... ARE NOT REPLACEMENTS!	201
FiNAL THOUGHTS	205
ACKNOWLEDGEMENTS	209
RECiPES	213
REFERENCES	227

DEDICATION

This book is dedicated to you.
May you live in happiness and health all the days of your life.

FOREWORD

There are two aspects to health and wellness: the food we choose and the nutrients it possesses; and how well our minds, bodies and spirit are able to take the foods we consume, digest it and nourish us as a whole. We are under such great challenges today in North America when it comes to understanding how to choose the right foods to fuel our body and our mind. Our soils are depleted, and conventional plants are weak and deficient. Plants aren't producing the antioxidants we desperately need and our bodies crave the nutrients we are lacking. We turn to highly-processed and artificially-colored foods with promised results printed on the pretty packages providing false hope they will quench our cravings and desires.

There has never been a greater state of an emergency than the silent catastrophe we are living today. Our body's ability to deal with stress is frayed, our ability to stay physically and mentally healthy has weakened, and our ability to think positively and stay focused has become fogged and blurred. We have become an overburdened, underappreciated, unhealthy, emotionally stressed out society. Just look at our crumbling healthcare system.

Throughout our lives we use food as the foundation for love, belonging, and comfort. The food industry knows how to tap in and create a false sense of hope keeping health-conscious shoppers hooked with the right marketing and packaging.

The confectionary, beverage and food industries know that our bodies have the ability to take in food and categorize it for later use based on not only nutrient content but also on reward and pleasure. The next time we are in a similar emotional state we will reach for the particular food based on related experiences. Just look at how big the snacking industry is.

When your body chemistry is balanced, you are balanced. Your body is getting all the nutrients it needs and you display emotions and behaviors that are in alignment with a healthy mind and body. You are better able to cope with stressful and emotional situations and attune to the positive outcome more readily. We are only scratching the surface on how our brain and gut are interconnected. Globally, more than 350 million people of all ages are suffering from depression and it affects approximately 14.8 million American adults aged 18 and older in a given year. More women are affected by depression than men, which may be the result of the intricate messaging of hormones throughout her lifetime. But how is our food affecting this delicate balance?

Hormones are special chemicals usually found in the glands of our endocrine system that release messengers directly into the blood and travel to the appropriate cells. Our cells then respond to the message. We only require microscopic amounts of hormones each day and this delicately balanced system requires the right nutrients. If nutrients are lacking, we end up with an unraveled communication system. Our cells and our hormones require the right nutrients from our food and are also affected by environmental factors, lifestyle including stress, and our outlook on life.

Look at the food consumed today. The SAD diet (Standard American Diet) contains genetically altered foods, grown in pesticide-laden nutrient-deficient soil, containing manipulated synthetic nutrients and chemical concoctions that numb senses and keep us coming back for more. These foods are so highly processed the finished products result in fillers, preservatives, additives, and extracts devoid of the vitamins, minerals and fatty acids, antioxidants, and probiotics we desperately need on a daily basis to keep our bodies and minds healthy. For good measure, the food industry adds on average four synthetic formulations of the naturally occurring 13 vitamins that were stripped away during the refinement process. How can we possibly stay healthy eating these types of foods that do not even meet our daily nutrient requirements?

So, what can we do? Remember, we have the ultimate choice. We need to get back to real unprocessed organic foods that are grown in the earth and feed off of the earth, naturally. This along with good digestion and supplementation will help us to nourish our body, brain, and our soul.

Vitamins and minerals along with good fats help normalize hormones and aid in supporting neurotransmitters.

Neurotransmitters help transmit our thoughts and direct our reactions to the behavior of others. We require fatty acids on a daily basis as we do not make them on our own. They are called "essential fatty acids" (EFAs) for a reason; they are essential to our body. Our nerves, brain, and thoughts require fatty acids, especially Omega 3 Fatty acids.

We now know from the mounting research that probiotics can help shape the integrity of our cells, hormones, and our brain function. We need polyphenol-rich foods to feed our microbiome on a daily basis. Due to depleted soils, we need quality supplementation in order to run our bodies and minds properly and to help us cope with our self-perpetuating stressful lives.

Everything that you are about to read in Devra's "Wake the Health Up" will open your mind and guide you along your path to wellness. The most wonderful part of Devra's journey is her openness to share it with you. If you thought you had to be perfect before getting healthy, or you think the author could not possibly understand what you are going through, think again. It is Devra's candidness that will spur you on in your journey to wellness.

Devra has endured traumatic experiences: the loss of loved ones, weight management her entire life, miscarriages, a daughter and husband who both survived cancer, holding the hands of her parents knowing she would have to let them go prematurely, succumbing way too early in life to preventable lifestyle diseases plaguing North Americans. Through it all

Devra, somehow, persevered. Instead of losing all faith, Devra turned to the power of her faith to spur her on.

Devra believed there had to be more to life than just pain, misery, cancer and ultimately dying too young. This intention of wonderment created a new universal path for Devra to follow; one that would lead her to her own health journey recovery, and ultimately, this book.

Once Devra got a taste of the "healthy side" she knew she was on to something. As Devra began to change her lifestyle along with her diet, she began to see the connections on how she was able to handle stress better and how the food choices directly impacted her health. Devra's healthier lifestyle gave her the confidence to bravely step out on her own and reinvent herself and her life.

This is when I first met Devra and her wonderful husband, Ray. Devra and Ray had come to Mexico for a week-long Health and Education Retreat in order to work on their own health while learning about nutrition and wellness to help others. With her Nutrition Advisor Certification in hand, Devra was inspired to learn more as she grew healthier and stronger.

Later, Devra took my training course in the USA, "Healthy Gut Advisor Home Training Program" that put the pieces all together. I have had the honor of teaching thousands the core concepts of nutrition, digestion, and healing.

When it comes to understanding emotions, physical endurance, and spiritual connection, it is food and the ability to digest it physically and emotionally that is the true key to health and wellness. This innate act allows for the nourishment of our cells, body, and soul. This gives us the strength to get through any difficulties allowing our bodies and minds to stay healthy and confident. Devra devoured the holistic teachings and it was an honor to have such an astute student thirsty for more in my programs.

With her second certificate, Devra was ready to take on the challenge of the Institute for Integrative Nutrition (IIN). Devra wanted to coach others and IIN was the final piece she needed.

With three certifications in less than five years, Devra is now coaching others how to experience the positive effects of good nutrition and supplementation so that they, too, can better navigate the perils of life's journey with confidence and positive outcomes. Devra has become a beacon of hope for those who think they can't be healthy even though they truly want to be. She knows what it is like to feel there is no hope. Devra is unstoppable.

I am simply amazed at Devra's tenacity to want more, not just for herself but for others. If she can feel this good, Devra knows everyone has the right to feel this good. With a book, "Wake the Health Up," an internet TV show; "Chew on This with Devra and Ray," and a podcast, "Wake the Health Up," Devra is tuning people in to wake the health up.

It is such an honor to have been given the gift to glimpse into Devra's life through her book. We truly do not know one another until we take the time to listen to their stories. Devra's story of loss was not the end of the road but merely the spark of her quest to want more. She cannot change what has happened in the past. She can learn from it and help shape the future of herself, her family and others who are willing to discover their path and take the journey to wellness.

We all have our difficult, painful pasts and we all have hopes, dreams, and desires that sometimes do not turn or manifest into what we were hoping. This is not an excuse to give up. There are times when you feel like you have no control, and that is the time when you must realize you are the control. We all have choices. Even if the choice we make is not the right one, we can make another choice to make it right. We must learn to never give up.

We need to learn how to tune into our own body and listen to what it is saying. When we are angry, sad, depressed or feeling low, this is the body communicating that something is out of alignment. Instead of listening, we reach for medications to treat the symptoms. Wake the Health Up! We do not have a medication deficiency.

We have come to this horrible misconception that if we are hormonal, we need medication. If we are sad, blue or depressed, we need medication. If we are fat, too thin, or just not right, there is a medication for that too. I promise you: never, ever...EVER will you have a deficiency of a medication. You could have a deficiency of B vitamins, Co-enzyme Q10 and magnesium that, when in good reserves, can make you feel more energetic and focused. Could you have a deficiency of essential fatty acids which can be treated with daily supplements so that hormones fall into balance, inflammation decreases, and you feel more balanced and centered? You bet!

As Devra would say; "Wake the Health Up!" We have to start tuning in and understanding how our nutritional needs impact our moods, behaviors, and our ability to cope. Devra is a prime example of how feeding her body the right nutrients allowed her to lose over fifty pounds. Not only has this boosted her confidence, it has also allowed her to reconnect with her energy and vitality. Devra is ebullient.

Epigenetics has proven that we are not governed by our genes, but rather our nutrition and external environmental influences. We need to Wake the Health Up and smell the nutrient-rich coffee alternatives and start taking responsibility for our own health.

Sure, we can all be dealt horrible experiences in our lives. And Devra is the prime example of the beautiful story of struggle and triumph and all the bumps and roadblocks that went along with it. Throughout her incredible life story, she honored her life's lessons in order to heal.

Many of us have forgotten that we too can change the situation we are in. Devra does an incredible job of reminding us of this crucial key component to wellness and health at any age. It is incredibly uncanny how Devra can be completely transparent about her journey in the hopes of helping another to step up and take responsibility. The most incredible journey you will ever take is the journey of YOU!

When Devra reflects back on her connection to food choices, what she was feeding her family along with what she has endured, she realized she needed answers and was prepared to implement the answers so that she could be around for a lifetime as a wife, mother, grandmother, and great-grandmother;

"As I seek answers to my questions, I have come to a fuller understanding of my own responsibility for the choices I make. Yes, genetics and environment may play a role in my health, but I'm responsible for understanding my options and making decisions to have the best possible life. And so are you."

Junk foods lead to junk thoughts and behaviors along with poor concentration, anger, grief, panic attacks, nervousness, unrest, feeling unloved, guilt, frustration, insecurity, restlessness, worry, crying spells, depression, fear, and phobias.

Whole foods from fruits, vegetables, nuts, seeds, whole grains, legumes, quality meat, and poultry lead to grounded positive thoughts and behaviors, including feeling full of life, happiness, feeling loved, good decision making, feeling connected, healthy, energetic, calm, intimate, eager to learn, grounded, alive, balanced and loved and, most of all, feeling and looking great with incredible energy and vitality at any age. Devra is proof of this.

Whatever it is that you are dealing with, I highly urge you to read Devra's recommendations. Keep this book with you because when you are ready to take the next step, Devra will be there to help you Wake the Health Up.

As Devra says, "It's your body. Love it or leave it. No one gets out of this life alive—every one of us will die—sooner or later. I prefer it to be later. Living here on earth or going home to glory are both a win. How you live—your quality of life—makes all the difference. The body is a magnificently designed machine, and it will support you in living out your dreams for your life when it is properly cared for."

Wake the Health Up will help you learn it is never too late to live a life of health and happiness and Devra is here to show you how.

Enjoy,

Karen Langston
CN, CNP, RNCP, NNCP, LE, LM
Founder of the Healthy Gut Advisor Home Study Program.
HealthyGutAdvisor.com

...A NOTE FROM THE AUTHOR

Habits formed over a lifetime inform and drive everything you think, say, and do, *unless* you make a conscious decision to do something differently at any given point in time.

Some habits are beneficial, and some habits derail you from your desired destination. Whatever you do won't get you where you want to go unless you have a roadmap. Just as it's imperative to know your values, goals, and vision in your personal and business relationships to get where you want to go, it's equally important for optimal health. If you, or I, aren't living in optimal health it's likely that we won't realize the full attainment of our life goals. If you have dreams, goals, and a vision for making your life and this world a better place, don't let poor health interfere. You can wake the health up and create optimal health for you and your family.

We get one body. One. We can steward our money, our time, and our resources, poorly or wisely. But if we don't become good stewards of the one body in which we dwell, then money, time, and resources will be the least of our concerns.

I'm grateful for each person (friend, author, speaker, colleague, coach) who challenges me to think differently about the choices I make and about my daily habits. Ultimately, I was challenged to analyze decisions that impacted my health. I was convicted by the way I abused, misused, neglected, and misunderstood the body in which I dwell. And I'm not alone. I see it happening across our nation.

This book is a result of years of reading, learning, and digesting information. My journey to intentionally improve my health began 12 years ago. I'm still on the journey. I want to share with you the things I wish I'd known—or acted on—years ago.

iNTRODUCTiON

I'm a woman who struggled with health and an unhealthy weight my entire life. I'm a woman who suffered through four miscarriages and then faced the devastating loss of our 3-day old son due to complications during childbirth. I'm a wife whose husband is a prostate cancer survivor. I'm a mother whose daughter is a cancer survivor. I'm a daughter who watched her parents live with debilitating symptoms and then watched them die prematurely as a result of complications from "lifestyle" diseases. I'm a friend who prayed with and cried with far too many friends who received a life-altering or life-ending diagnosis for themselves or a loved one. I'm a grandmother and great-grandmother concerned about the present and future health of all children born in this age.

As a result of such experiences, I became deeply curious about what may be at the root of my own health issues and the apparent escalation of diseases that have impacted and continue to impact those I love.

The United States is the wealthiest country in the world with advanced medical knowledge, yet many people in the United

States of America are malnourished *and* obese. A multitude of serious diseases that affect human life is on the rise. And I wonder why. Do you wonder why?

Here are a few other things that cause me to wonder:
- I wonder why food-like stuff created in a lab and void of nutritional value is sold as food.
- I wonder why known toxins such as mercury, fluoride, and glyphosate, are allowed into our bodies and our environment.
- I wonder why food dyes and other additives that increasingly show harm and behavior change still show up in food—especially food commercially targeted to children.
- I wonder why some companies manufacture and distribute foods without genetically modified organisms (GMOs) to other countries with higher standards, yet they market GMO versions in the United States.
- I wonder why companies spend millions and millions of dollars to prevent labeling laws if there is no problem with GMO food.
- I wonder why, despite the U.S. having the most advanced "health" care system in the world, infectious diseases have been replaced by a rise in degenerative or lifestyle diseases. We're not dying later—we're dying longer.

I don't have all the answers. But I do have a lot of questions. The answers can typically be found in the questions we ask. The more I question, the more I wonder. And the wondering stirs a thirst within me to do my own research in search of answers. The more I learn and read from the experts, the more curious I become and the more questions I have. I hope you'll become curious along with me.

As I seek answers to my questions, I have come to a fuller understanding of my own responsibility for the choices I make. Yes, genetics and environment may play a role in my health, but I'm responsible for understanding my options and making decisions to have the best possible life. And so are you.

Before I began this journey, I took the food I fed my family at face value. Food is food, right? The body and hair products I used were safe, right? If a product was on a store shelf then surely it was safe for consumption, right?

I was a slow adopter of many of the topics covered in this book. I didn't understand their impact on my health. I was a doubter until I was confronted with my own health issues. I thought if I covered my eyes and ears to the growing evidence, then I didn't have to acknowledge that I had to take responsibility for my health. I am the one ultimately responsible for my health. As my curiosity led to learning, I came to realize that ignorance is NOT bliss. Uninformed is unarmed. I couldn't assume anyone else had my best health in mind when making, creating, marketing, and distributing products for me to buy.

"Wake up and smell the coffee" and wonder in what way coffee benefits you. Does drinking coffee support your health or does coffee undermine your health? Does eating junk food support your health or does it undermine your health? Does drinking water support your health or does it undermine your health? Does it matter if you don't drink water? Do the "healthy" products you buy for your children support health, or undermine health? You must wake up and pay attention to what supports your health. The answers begin with a question.

I encourage you to wonder. I want to inspire you to do your own research—not a quick Google search to affirm your current point of view. Search a variety of reputable sources. Then make informed decisions that best support your own health and wellbeing, and that of your loved ones.

These days, there are specialists and experts on both sides of most medical and environmental issues who can show clear evidence about why their scientific study or opinion is the truth—or why the opposing viewpoint is flawed. There are multiple points of view on virtually *every* health topic. The battle rages on about the causes of autism and other behavioral or mental disorders like depression, ADHD, etc. The battle rages on between vaccines as a miracle and vaccines as a potential cause of injury. The battle rages on about the effects of pesticides, herbicides, and fungicides in and on the food supply and to what degree they affect the human body. I don't know about you, but it makes my head spin.

It takes time to research and sort out the information. But it is crucial for you to do so. If you don't take time to understand how to create a healthier you, you'll likely have to take time to deal with the consequences of an unhealthy you.

Regardless of the sometimes divisive and conflicting expert opinions, there are actions you can take—habits you can develop—to help the body you live in to be the healthiest body possible.

> THE PROBLEM WITH THE WORLD IS NOT THAT PEOPLE KNOW TOO LITTLE, BUT THAT THEY KNOW SO MANY THINGS THAT AREN'T SO.
> – MARK TWAIN

It's your body. Love it or leave it. No one gets out of this life alive—every one of us will die—sooner or later. I prefer it to be later. Living here on earth or going home to glory are both a win. However, how you live—your quality of life—makes all the difference. The body is a magnificently designed machine, and it will support you in living out your dreams for your life when it is properly cared for.

Wake the Health Up

MY JOURNEY

I struggled with illness and excess weight my entire life. I began to develop my food and lifestyle behaviors at a very young age. I wasn't necessarily an overeater as a child. My parents made an effort to prepare balanced meals. Breakfast was often cereal, lunch was peanut butter and jelly or a bologna sandwich, and dinner was meat, starch, canned veggie, and a salad. That was the standard American diet at that time. I don't recall having a bunch of snacks in our home. We didn't get much candy. We didn't eat out very often. We'd go to the NCO club (a restaurant on an Air Force base) occasionally. McDonald's was a coveted treat. I loved McDonald's as a young child and now, just seeing the Golden Arches triggers special memories of our family trips to McDonald's. I was very young when I began to equate reward, treat, and love—to food.

My parents loved to dance—swing, square, jitterbug—but I always felt like I had two left feet, so I watched as they danced. I couldn't run very fast, so I didn't run at all. I couldn't manage the monkey bars, so I stopped trying. I couldn't keep up with my classmates at recess, so I stopped trying and retreated into a world of books. I fell in love with reading. I could escape into a world of adventure and intrigue where good always triumphed. As a young child and preteen, I laid on my backside and read all the children's classics I could devour. Play, sports, and outdoor activity took a backseat—a far back seat—to the world of adventure found in the printed word. When I look at my childhood pictures, I see *now* that I was just slightly "bigger" than the other kids. But I heard the words chubby, baby fat, and, big-boned used to describe me, and I gave those words room in my head.

> IT ISN'T THAT THEY CAN'T SEE THE SOLUTION. IT IS THAT THEY CAN'T SEE THE PROBLEM.
> — G.K. CHESTERTON

When I was 14, my dad transferred to Ramey Air Force Base in Puerto Rico. The good news was that I had to walk everywhere. The bad news was that my self-image had already become warped. The view I had of myself and the picture caught by the camera were utterly different. I understand that now. It was the late 1960's and the famous ultra-skinny model, Twiggy, was "the" role model for modern fashion—and I was no Twiggy! And so, the story I claimed was that I was fat. The story I told myself at the time was that to be of value, loved, liked, or to be accepted I must be skin and bones like Twiggy. By the time I was 15, I had begun the revolving door of fad diets and drinking diet sodas to achieve the ideal of a "perfect" me. But, I never got "skinny!"

I married at a very young age. My husband had a very healthy attitude about food—except he did love desserts. Can you say dessert for breakfast, lunch, and dinner? I learned to make some incredibly delicious desserts. My fascination with fad diets ceased for a time. For many years my weight remained stable, and I was reasonably healthy—except for recurring urinary tract infections treated with a round of antibiotics two or three times a year.

But, by the time I was about 35 I had gained 60 pounds. Some of it I acquired during five failed pregnancies. In desperation to lose weight, I began to experiment with every new diet that came along: the Atkins Diet, the Cabbage Soup Diet, Weight Watchers, TOPS (Taking Off Pounds Sensibly), and an 800-calorie diet. You name it, and I most likely tried it. Despite the temporary success, I quickly "found" the weight I had lost. None of the "diets" that seemed to be successful for my friends, or the people on the cover of the magazines, worked for me.

About this time a doctor encouraged me to:
- drink diet soda in place of regular soda and sweet tea.
- remove sugar from my diet and replace it with aspartame.
- restrict *all* fat and use margarine in its place.

And I followed my doctor's orders. While consuming non-fat, sugar-free, artificial sweeteners, fake butter products, and drinking diet coke, the scale climbed an *additional 40 pounds*. I also developed a seizure disorder. I was frustrated and ill-informed. Turns out, so was my doctor.

As those pounds began to pile on my self-esteem hit bottom. The verbal abuse in my head roared with thoughts like: I'm stupid, I'm fat, I can't do anything right.

I blamed myself. I SHOULD be able to stop eating. The more I listened to the negative voices, the more I beat myself up and adopted a very unhealthy attitude about food. Can you relate?

I coped with the confidence-draining weight gain, and my inability to control my weight and the devastating life events that seemed to just keep coming, the only way I knew how. I shoved my feelings down and covered them with food. My faith was always solid because I had enough evidence in my life that God was present and at work despite my circumstances. Life happens. It's all about how we deal with it. However, I'm not sure I ever dealt with *it*.

It was the baby who died in childbirth. *It* was four miscarriages. *It* was my husband's cancer and the recurring complications. *It* was my beloved daughter's battle with drug addiction. *It* was my mom's devastating illness that claimed her life far too young. Whatever the "*it*" was, I shoved my feelings and emotions deep and smacked on a happy face. What I didn't understand at the time was the impact the unresolved pain and anger, coupled with the nutritional deficiencies in my diet, and all that negative self-talk had on my declining health.

Then one day, seemingly out-of-the-blue, my body revolted with a violent gallbladder attack which required emergency removal of my gallbladder.

After the surgery, I learned that my gallbladder was gangrenous. How does that even happen? My body had been giving me warning signs for years. I didn't recognize the warning signs. Even after the experience with my gallbladder, I neglected other warning signs. I was oblivious to the fact that these symptoms were signs that something was awry in my body.

By the time I was 51, I was a physical mess. Every sniffle that walked past me, or germ that lingered on a doorknob, I adopted and took home and nurtured. I had three to four severe bouts of bronchitis a year, each lasting three or four weeks at a time. That was four months of misery, year in and year out. My immune system was shot!

I continued to struggle with an unhealthy weight along with extreme fatigue, high blood pressure, metabolic syndrome, intestinal problems, depression, recurring yeast and bladder infections, and the seizure disorder. The anti-seizure medication left me in a fog. I lived on antibiotics. I ate a standard American diet (SAD). Fast food was a treat—*a daily one*, and sometimes even twice a day because it was so darn cheap. Oh, I liked salads, loaded with ranch dressing and fake bacon bits. Other than romaine and iceberg lettuce and spinach occasionally, fresh leafy greens rarely passed my lips. Even though I felt miserable most of the time, I kept going, and I continued to burn the candle at both ends. I had convinced myself that sleep was a necessary evil and I grudgingly allowed myself five or six hours of sleep a night—sometimes. My favorite saying was "I can sleep when I'm dead!" I didn't understand the vital role of sleep. Little did I realize that if I didn't get adequate sleep, death could come much sooner.

The most valuable asset you and I have is our health. I didn't understand that until I almost lost my health entirely.

My doctor cautioned me that if something didn't change soon, I was facing diabetes and heart disease. The same diseases that eventually claimed the lives of my parents prematurely. My mother died at the age of 61 from complications of diabetes. She also struggled with achieving a healthy weight her entire life. Her mother before her also had diabetes. My grandmother called it "sugar." I may have the genetic code for diabetes, but now I wonder if I was pre-diabetic because diabetes *ran in my family,* or if was I pre-diabetic because I learned my eating habits and lifestyle behaviors from my parents. With this warning from my doctor, I did try to do better. However, I was still frustrated and ill-informed. Nothing I tried seemed to work.

I remember praying, "I just want to know how to feel 'normal' once more!" God answered my prayers. The first answer came as a result of a chance conversation after a Toastmaster's meeting. I was invited to attend a personal growth & development weekend event. As a result of that weekend, I realized that I clung to belief systems about myself, the world around me, and my place in it that were preventing me from making positive changes in my life. I had some "growing up" to do. I discovered that I could choose to be a victim of life's circumstances or I could choose to take responsibility for my life, and my responses to events in my life. I began to process the pain and suffering I thought I had tucked away so neatly. I started to understand the power of the thoughts, words, and images I used and the role they played in my overall wellbeing. I decided to only speak words that lifted my spirit up. And most importantly, I decided to see myself through God's eyes.

I had to change my story. The story was killing me in more ways than one. In response to the pain and depression I faced in my life, the words and events interpreted by a young child that lay deep in my subconscious were given power. Words like: You don't matter. You should be seen and not heard. If I wanted your opinion, I'd tell you. Who do you think you are? Don't speak unless spoken to. I'm not even aware of when or where I initially heard those words, but when my mental, physical, and spiritual defenses were down I gave those words power in my life. We all accumulate bad impactful experiences—things people have said to us or done to us—consciously or subconsciously. Eventually, they can manifest in physical illnesses unless we address them.

Choices made by other people also impacted the chapters of my life. But the only person who can write how my life story unfolds—is me. The only person who ultimately writes your story is you. We write our story through the decisions we make, by the attitudes we adopt in response to what happens to us, and by how we choose to live out our story.

The second answer to my prayer came via an introduction to a pharmaceutical grade supplement company. The products had a positive impact on my health. In a short period, I felt a significant difference. Once my body began receiving the nutrients it sorely needed, it could start the repair process. I quickly released 40 pounds, had more clarity, and more energy. My experience using those supplements triggered my interest in the connection between nutrition and health.

I began eating healthier, but some of my food choices were still negatively impacting my health. And the weight release came to a standstill. I didn't understand. Despite healthier eating habits and using high-quality supplements several symptoms including excess weight persisted. Of course, I was still burning the candle at both ends. I didn't manage stress well. I foolishly convinced myself that I worked best under pressure and that sleep was overrated. I later learned about the relevance of quality sleep, its impact on the body, and the consequence of sleep deprivation. I learned that the healthy food I was eating wasn't healthy for me. I discovered I had a leaky gut and a host of related health issues. I needed answers to these questions: What is leaky gut? What causes a leaky gut and how on earth could I get rid of it? Was a leaky gut connected to my medical problems?

I was mentally and physically healthier, but it was clear I still had some changes to make to achieve optimal health.

As I learned, I continued to change my food and lifestyle behaviors. I no longer live with seizures or chronic bronchitis. My digestive issues are healing, and my immune system can ward off most colds and flu viruses. Now, in my 60's, I'm healthier and happier than I was in my 30's.

As a result of my health journey and recovery, I'm more and more curious about how the human body functions as one whole. The health issues my loved ones experienced stirred that curiosity. To satisfy my curiosity, I began to read, study, and learn. The more I learned, the more I wondered about what creates health and what causes disease in the body. I can be a slow learner. Biology wasn't my favorite subject in high school. That was then. Now, I love biology—especially human biology.

I took an online course (Healthy Gut Advisor Weekend Intensive training) with Karen Langston, Holistic Nutritionist, and then I became a student at the Institute of Integrative Nutrition, and I continue to read, research, and study health-related topics because I want to be a resource for people praying for their own "norm." I now challenge the concept of normal in today's health landscape. Normal isn't always natural. Normal, or the norm, is just what we have come to accept. I now seek optimal health as my new normal. I'm thankful that my parents' health challenges don't have to become my reality. I'm grateful for the wake-up call to examine the story I was telling myself about my health and my worth and that my health story could be re-written. I'm grateful for what I have learned and for my restored and still improving health.

Wake the Health Up

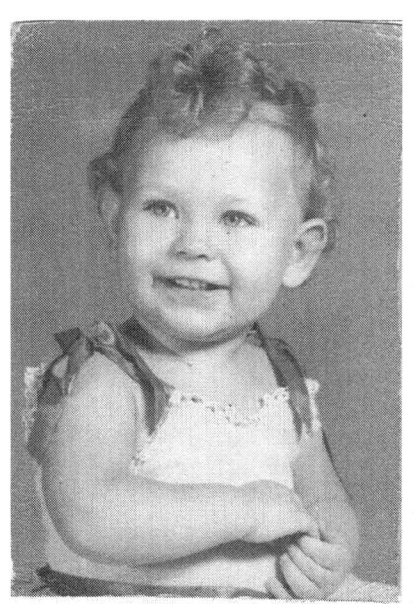
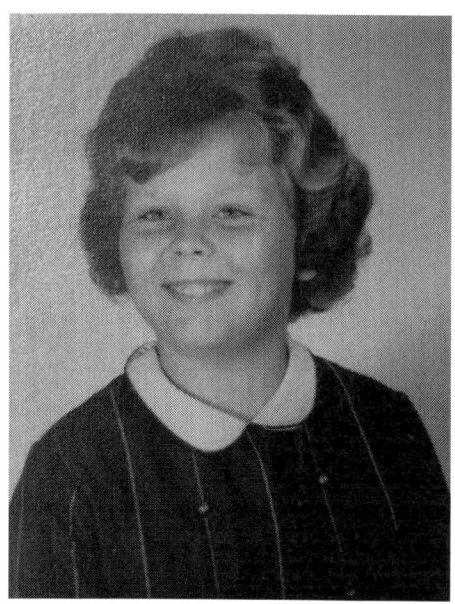
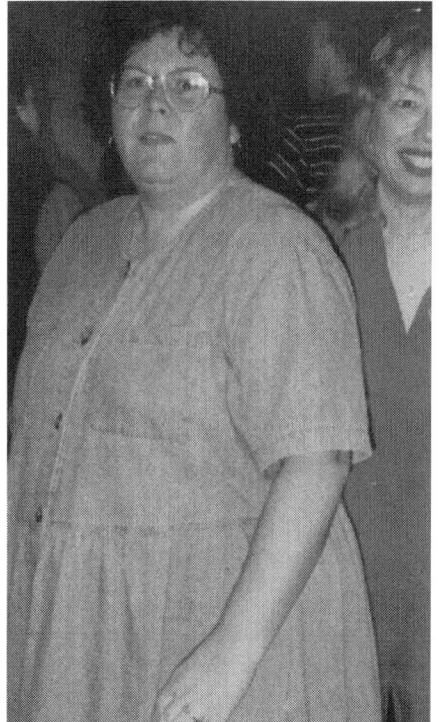
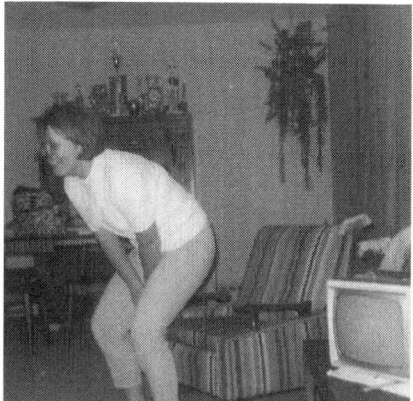
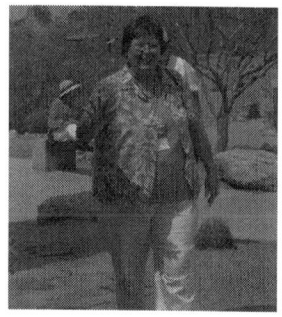

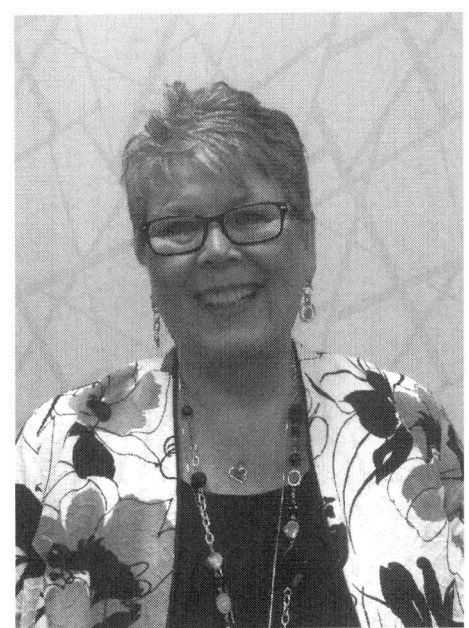
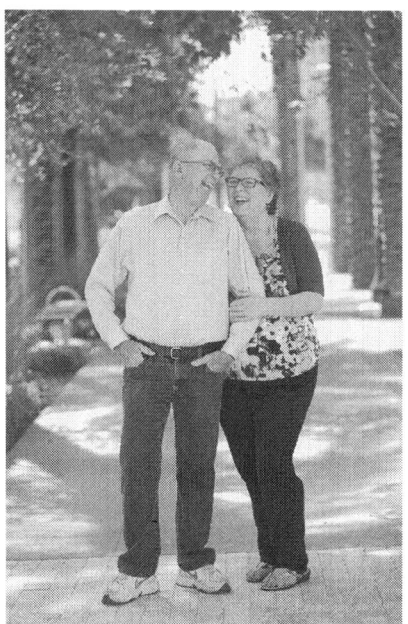
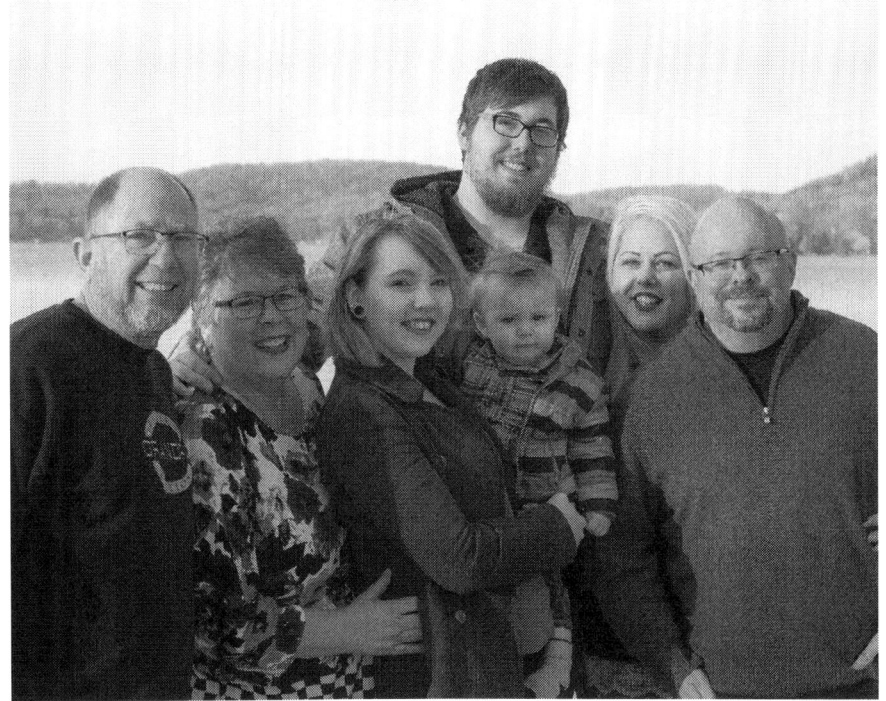

Wake the Health Up

WHAT DO *YOU* WANT?

I was blessed to serve on a church staff for 16 years. It was a joy to witness people discover and employ their passions and gifts in ministry. However, over the years many faithful servants lived with symptoms or were diagnosed with illnesses that prevented them from serving and from living life to its fullest. Their spirit was willing, but the body was weak and getting weaker—and sicker. Even those who seemed to live a healthy lifestyle, eat well, and exercise received devastating life-altering diagnoses. And some also died.

All too often in our society symptoms are accepted as normal. Acceptance sounds like, "I'm getting older; I guess I should expect to get _____" (fill in the blank); "Disease is inevitable." "I will die of something."

Some even question if the illness is a punishment. These questions arise, "What did I do to deserve this?" Or, "Why is God punishing me?" Blaming God is easy.

What if God doesn't have anything to do with the *cause* of your illness? What if sickness and disease are conditions of living in an imperfect world? What if the diagnosis is a result of personal lifestyle choices? What if the environment you live in plays a role? What if the quality of food, air, and water are the culprits?

Taking responsibility for your health doesn't mean you'll avoid illness. There are too many factors that can affect the overall quality of your health. Even people who appear healthy—eat well, exercise, etc.—get cancer.

Death *is* inevitable. What I'm more concerned with is the *quality* of life we have while we're still living. I wonder if aches, pains, and illnesses have to be inevitable. Do they? People say, "I want to feed the homeless (or travel, or play golf, or…) but I can't because my back hurts." Or, "My stomach hurts." or, "I have migraines." or, "My joints don't work—they hurt!" Or, "I just can't get enough sleep." Or, "I have cancer." Even though we "hate" cancer and everything else from acne to reflux, joint pains, autism, ADHD, diabetes, autoimmune disease, and allergies, we continue to accept them as normal or inevitable. It seems we have come to expect and accept these diseases as a normal part of living. What if that need not be true? What if "normal" isn't necessarily "natural?" What if what we consider normal is actually abnormal?

The human body has a magnificent, intricate design. A healthy body can support, defend, and heal itself. It must be given proper care and nutrition to function optimally—the way it was designed to operate. Every part of the human body connects to every other part of the body. When one part of the body is injured, every other part of the body is affected. Have you ever stubbed your toe? I have too, and more than my toe reacts to the pain. Likewise, small symptoms in one part of the body are a sign that something isn't right somewhere in the body. Chronic illness doesn't just appear on the day of diagnosis. The human body will present clues, sometimes for decades before diagnosis. Yet, often we misread the warning signs as symptoms related to only getting older. Your body is speaking to you. Wake the health up! It's time to pay attention.

We seem to take for granted the body in which we dwell—until it starts to break down. Every person is uniquely designed and gifted for a purpose, and if we're angry, irritable, moody, achy, or downright sick, we can't embrace our full potential and do what we were created to do.

I have studied to unearth answers about how to live a healthy life. And I have more questions. It's not as simple as it once was to be healthy. We're advised to put down the fork, eat healthier, and to exercise more—sounds simple enough. So why is it so hard to do? Eating healthy is complicated these days. "Healthy" is more than choosing the quantity of food on your plate or skipping dessert.

And what about exercise? How much should you exercise—how much is enough or too much? Should it be weight-bearing? Is walking enough exercise? Do you need to spend to an hour at the gym each day? Can't "exercise;" what do you do? Don't let questions stop you. Let them push you toward the answers that lead to improved health.

Wake the Health Up

YOUR JOURNEY BEGINS HERE

I ask you to consider these questions:

1. Are you as healthy as you want to be?
2. Do you have the mental clarity to accomplish your daily tasks?
3. Do you have the physical agility to do what you love to do?
4. Are you sick and tired, or downright lethargic all the time?
5. Do you have allergies?
6. Do you have little aches and pains that hold you back—just a bit?
7. Do symptoms immobilize you way too often?
8. Do you routinely sleep through the night?
9. Have you forgotten what joy and vitality feel like?
10. Are you ready for a lifestyle overhaul?

What if small, simple changes in daily habits could make a significant difference in your overall wellbeing and your vitality? They can. Complacency isn't the answer! You're reading this book, so it's likely you want to make changes to improve your life. The time to start making changes is now!

Maybe you consider yourself reasonably healthy right now. You can eat what you want, and nothing seems to "bother" you. Keeping in mind that disease rarely manifests overnight, will your current eating and lifestyle habits promote the healthy life you want to have in one or even 50 years from now?

If not, what are you willing to change? You have personal habits and behaviors that you must adjust to minimize their harm and maximize their benefit.

Can you relate to this common scenario? You wake up ready to take on the day and crush your business goals, your health goals, your family commitments—and finish the big project before the deadline. You make it to 10 am, and then you spot the box of goodies in the break room. The little voice in your head whispers "Go ahead, you deserve it." Or, "Just one won't hurt." A colleague, friend, or family member echoes the voice in your head. "Oh, come on! Just one won't hurt!" And despite your very best intentions, you snatch something out of that box thinking "Just this once…" and down it goes. Then, the moment you finish licking your lips of whatever yummy was in that box, shame sets in. In discouragement, you pick up the emotional bat and start beating yourself up. That little voice whispers: "Well, you already screwed up your diet today, you might as well eat whatever you want now, and start tomorrow." And letting yourself off the hook for the whole day, you grab *just one more* and head back to your project.

If you choose to indulge in whatever temptations hang out in the break room, (or your kitchen pantry) put the bat away and stop beating yourself up over one choice. You have not ruined the whole day. Now, there are reasons why eating the first one creates an intense craving for another and another and we will talk about that in a later chapter. But for now, give yourself some grace.

Seek to make small changes. Aim for progress. Don't expect perfection right away—if ever. Give up the all or nothing notion. It doesn't serve you.

Love yourself—your body—and feed it well. If you feel like you need a treat, choose one that will support your health goals—not dismantle them. Don't use "treats" to sabotage your goals. You deserve to be your healthiest self. *However,* if you do choose to eat candy, cake, or a sugary treat change the narrative. Don't choose to have the "treat" because you deserve it and don't beat yourself up after you eat it. Enjoy the heck out of the "treat" and then make a different choice—that better supports your health—the rest of the day.

It's necessary to celebrate success—even the smallest victories—because the victories combine to make a huge difference. Decide right now what you'll reach for and *how* you'll reward yourself when you reach for a treat. Maybe with a small piece of dark chocolate. Perhaps a glass of wine at the end of the week. Perhaps a homemade cookie or dessert made with high-quality ingredients. Or, maybe your "treat" will be a long walk, a soak in the bath, or a massage. The "treat" doesn't need to be food related. Planning ahead is essential. How will you celebrate your successes?

Each person has the power to choose a healthier lifestyle. In seeking a healthier lifestyle, some choices you make might cause more harm than good. What you don't know CAN hurt you. It's difficult to fix what is standing between you and your health goals if you aren't even aware what the culprits might be. We must wake up to the health care crisis that's consuming us individually and as a nation. Wake the health up to those things that are at the root of the crisis. My journey has brought me to a full-blown passion for educating others. I'm compelled to share why it's crucial to nurture and care for our bodies *before* faced with a devastating diagnosis.

Lifestyle, poor dietary habits, lack of movement, negative thought processes, and even environmental toxins can leave you feeling sickly, sluggish, achy, and even depressed. Cleaning up the food you eat, the air you breathe, the water you drink, and the thoughts you think can increase your energy, balance your hormones, and improve your mood. Even though environmental toxins play a role in health, personal responsibility and developing proactive lifestyle habits gives you a critical health advantage.

Healthy habits go beyond the food you eat. Virtually everything you consume, think, and do (or don't do) fosters health—or disease. How you choose to care for your body, your mind, and your spirit has an impact on your energy, vitality, and overall health. Everyone has the potential to have a healthier life.

Become the healthiest you; a healthier you not only benefits you, it benefits us all.

As you begin this journey, be kind to yourself. Love yourself! Loving yourself includes sleep, self-care, and the proper care and feeding of the human body. Part of your health journey is the story you tell yourself. If you have a habit of beating yourself up when you make a choice that's not in your best interest, stop it!

The story we tell ourselves is often rooted in how we see ourselves and how we see ourselves is rooted in how we processed what others say or have said to us over the years. The words we speak to ourselves are significant as well. Your brain can't tell the difference between real or imagined. Believing negative stories makes them your reality. Luckily, we can take control of our stories by training our minds to notice and replace these negative stories with positive thoughts.

A positive mindset in your health journey is vital to your optimal health. The average person has an estimated 70,000 thoughts per day! Take a moment to think about the thoughts that run through your mind. Are they positive and uplifting? "Today is an amazing day!" Or are they negative, self-defeating, or self-deprecating? "I am not good enough."

Pessimistic thoughts and words create a domino effect of negativity in your life. Optimistic thoughts can boost your mood, your spirit, and generate even more positivity and happiness in your life. Your thoughts affect how you live and how others perceive you. The good news is you don't have to live with negative mental chatter. Choose to change the thought channel and allow only positive, uplifting thoughts, words, and actions to flow into and through you. You have complete choice in how you'll react in any given moment. Practice cultivating a happy outlook.

What story are you telling yourself? What words do you give power to? How is the story you're telling yourself impacting your health? If you're going to tell yourself a story—make sure it's a positive one!

> ONCE A PERSON IS DETERMINED TO HELP THEMSELVES, THERE IS NOTHING THAT CAN STOP THEM.
> — NELSON MANDELA

Take a few minutes right now and complete this short exercise.

1. Close your eyes for a moment and take a deep breath. Become aware of how your body feels at this very moment.
2. How do you feel? How is your energy level? What symptoms plague you? Write them down.
3. Now write down your intentions for reading this book. What caused you to purchase this book? What do you hope to learn?
4. Are you ready to make changes in your lifestyle and habits?
5. Now, picture yourself feeling clear-minded, energetic and ready to take on anything. What will you feel like by giving your body, mind, and spirit the proper care and feeding? What will you be able to do? What do you see? Write it down in vivid detail.

Wake the Health Up

MiNDSET—WHERE CHANGE BEGiNS

As you begin to take small steps and create new habits, they will affect significant change and impact your health for *good*. Change can be easy, or change can be hard. You choose. Some change comes in an instant; you decide to change, and something deep within you complies, and you make a shift. Was there a time in your life when that happened? What triggered the decision to change? Was the change temporary or long-lasting?

I've known people with a 3-pack-a-day smoking habit. They laid down the cigarettes one day and never smoked another. My mother was one of those people. I begged her for years to stop smoking. As a child, I'd even throw her cigarettes away. That didn't go over well! But one day, she laid them down, walked away, and never smoked again. Something similar happened to me with diet soda. I "knew" I should stop drinking it. I wanted to stop drinking it (sort of). I was addicted to the fizz—I LOVED the fizz. I was addicted to the caffeine. I was addicted to the sweet taste. I was addicted to the habit. I was addicted to the free supersize. I was addicted! It was hard to give it up. I'll admit that it took several years for me to stop drinking diet anything.

I don't even remember the final straw that prompted me to quit. Maybe it was opening my eyes to my declining health and continual weight gain. Perhaps it was the articles I read that pointed to the danger of sugar substitutes and how they contributed to weight gain and dozens of other health-related symptoms. Even though I learned about the reported risks of sugar substitutes, it was *hard* to quit. And it can be hard to manage the continued struggle with sugar. But the impact diet sodas and sugar have on my body is *hard* as well. Life is much easier without them.

You can choose the mindset that "it" is hard. And it will be hard. Determine what *it* is that you what to change and then focus on the outcome you want. Imagine how you'll feel once you make the change? Living with annoying symptoms, illness, and disease is hard, especially when your condition prevents you from doing what you want to do. Changing lifestyle behaviors can be hard—or not—depending on your mindset. It's up to you to choose *which* hard you want to live with.

When you decide to make positive changes, a transformation will happen as you consistently put into practice a new way of thinking and creating healthy habits. Be kind to yourself in the process. Give yourself grace. It took your whole life to arrive where you are today. There is no quick fix.

Use a journal and track your daily progress each night for the next 28 days and ask yourself these questions at the end of each day.
1. What went well?
2. What were your challenges?
3. What were your triggers?
4. What is your plan for tomorrow? What will you do differently?

> i HAVE CHOSEN To BE HAPPY
> BECAUSE iT iS GOOD FOR MY HEALTH.
> – VOLTAIRE

Wake the Health Up

THE ROOT OF iT!

When it comes to chronic disease, the current Western health care system, in many cases, merely offers bandages in the form of prescriptions and over-the-counter medications that mask symptoms instead of seeking out and correcting the source of the inflammation, or the root cause of the disease or illness. If you want to create optimal health, you must change the way you think about health, health care, and disease.

Each year, tens of billions of dollars are spent on medical research and development. Nearly a hundred billion dollars has been spent over the past 45 years to fight the war on cancer by the National Cancer Institute alone. Despite the vast sums of money spent treating and/or researching cures for heart disease, obesity, ADHD, autism, cancer, type 2 diabetes, and more than 100 other autoimmune conditions they continue to exist. (1) They don't just "exist," they are on the rise!

According to the National Center for Chronic Disease Prevention and Health Promotion (an office of the CDC), "one in two adults in the US has a chronic disease and one in four adults has two or more." (2). Chronic diseases and the conditions that lead to them are considered lifestyle diseases. Meaning, they're preventable! (3)

The CDC also states "86% of the nation's $2.7 trillion in annual health care expenditures are for people with chronic and mental health conditions." (4) Chronic diseases are generally defined as conditions lasting one year or more, limit daily activities, and require ongoing medical attention. Chronic disease includes:

- Alzheimer's Disease
- Arthritis
- Breast Cancer
- Cervical Cancer
- Colorectal/Colon Cancer
- Chronic Obstructive Pulmonary Disease (COPD)
- Depression
- Diabetes (I, II)
- Epilepsy
- Gynecologic Cancer
- Heart Disease
- High Blood Pressure
- Kidney Disease
- Obesity
- Pre-diabetes
- Prostate Cancer
- Skin Cancer
- Stroke

Children are also being diagnosed with many of these diseases at increasing rates. One-fourth of children in the US 2-8 years of age have a chronic health condition, including diabetes (type 1 and type 2), allergies, ADHD, autism, behavioral issues, cancer, and other autoimmune diseases. (5) And these numbers are on the rise.

Chronic inflammation is the root cause of most diseases. (6)

What if we, individually and as a nation, invested more time, money, and energy on preventing inflammation instead of waiting on an elusive cure? What if you consider, for just a moment, that you don't need to wait for a drug company, or the government, or the food suppliers, or anyone else to act responsibly and instead take personal responsibility? What if you begin today with your own resources and your body's own wisdom to avert a dreaded diagnosis in one year or 30 years? You don't wake up one day and suddenly develop cancer, heart disease, or even acne. What if you take action today to create a healthier lifestyle? What if you can reduce the inflammation and live the most robust life possible?

> **AN OUNCE OF PREVENTION IS WORTH A POUND OF CURE.**
> – BENJAMIN FRANKLIN

"An ounce of prevention is worth a pound of cure." (7) When Benjamin Franklin penned this in the 1700's, he wasn't referring to health. He was referring to fire dangers. However, this sentiment can be applied to any aspect of your personal life, and it's especially true when it comes to long-term health.

Navigating life can be stressful. People are busy going to college, getting a job, climbing the corporate ladder, building a business, raising kids, commuting, working, running to sports practice and after-school activities, volunteering in the community and in church, and squeezing in exercise, and study—or not. Finding the best way to feed yourself and your family is a challenge. Maybe you think you're doing the best you can. But what if your best in one area of your life is compromising your best in another area—your health? While busy trying to survive, unintentional consequences arise.

Most parents wouldn't intentionally hurt their child. A reasonable person wouldn't knowingly consume poison, and yet makes decisions every day that expose loved ones to harmful factors that can have a negative impact on health and wellbeing. The challenge is that the harm isn't always immediate—you don't see it or feel it right away—it doesn't yell DANGER! WARNING! The damage may be slow, cumulative, and hidden in the symptoms many have come to accept as normal. These symptoms lead to chronic disease or premature death if ignored.

There is a health crisis going on around us. The crisis isn't just the state of health insurance or health care. The crisis has its roots in the choices we make and in our own behaviors. What?!?!?

Back to my story. I thought I was making good choices to improve my health. I was eating whole grains, whole wheat, diet sodas, low fat, and low carb. In addition to eating food that was actually compromising my health, I wasn't sleeping, and I embraced stress in my life. I was sick, getting fatter, and my energy was non-existent. I realized I wasn't alone. What was happening? I realized I didn't understand what it meant to eat healthily or to be healthy. Do you?

If we don't wake up and pay attention to what is being done to our food, water, and air supply, our "good" choices may not result in good health.

In today's world, self-proclaimed experts line up on both sides of virtually every topic on every media and social media outlet. There are countless books, podcasts, webinars, magazines, cookbooks, and top Google searches about how to be healthy. All this information can be confusing, conflicting, and even misleading—especially concerning health and wellness—and it's time-consuming to study it. But your long-term health and the health of your family are worth it. Do your research. Question everything. Read more than one opinion and read with an open mind. Be curious about what is at the root of your health issues and question everything, even those things you think you know. Remember, what you don't know CAN hurt you.

What if prevention could be the best cure? Become an informed consumer and then take whatever action you can to create a healthier lifestyle for you and your family. Your life depends on it!

There is good news. Most experts do agree that increasing whole leafy greens, getting adequate sleep, reducing or managing stress, staying hydrated, and improving the immune system all play a role in improved health. YOU have total control over how to improve these behaviors.

This is a wake-up call for you. You have but one body. Every human body requires proper care and feeding of the mind, body, and spirit to thrive in optimal health. It's up to you!

My objective for writing this book is to encourage you, even beg you, to wake up and to question what is impacting your health today, your long-term health, and the health of your family.

This book is designed to help you create transformational change. It can help you navigate the health and wellness information jungle and help you choose what steps you will take to improve your health.

This book is designed to help you create transformational change. It can help you navigate the health and wellness information jungle and help you choose what steps you will take to improve your health.

As you discover what may be interfering with your ability to live life healthy, happy, and whole, you can begin to make informed decisions acted out in small, simple changes. Those simple changes will lead to lifelong habits and a transformation in your long-term health—for you and your loved ones. Remember that the synergy that occurs when multiple changes are introduced can be impressive. Likewise, continuing poor health habits in one or more areas may lessen the effects of a positive difference in another.

As you implement the action steps in this book and make them habits, you'll be on the road to a healthier you. Your future self will be eternally grateful. Get ready for a lifestyle overhaul, a fresh mind, and a revitalized body.

It's time to wake the health up. Begin today! Nourish your mind, body, and spirit with what you choose to consume, do, think, and buy. As we do this together, we can change the health of our nation, our communities, our families, and ourselves.

Wake the Health Up

IT'S GENETIC! IS IT THAT SIMPLE?

Your genetic blueprint was formed at the moment of conception. However, your genetic predisposition isn't a reason to live as if you're destined to develop a condition.

Diabetes runs in my family. I have a genetic disposition to develop diabetes. But what if the WAY I learned to eat and move my body has more to do with the expression of diabetes than my genes do? What if what I choose to eat and how I choose to live determines what inherited genes are expressed and which lie dormant?

A relatively new field of study—epigenetics—is revealing how factors such as diet, stress, lifestyle behaviors, and environmental conditions can impact gene expression in the body; in most cases, genes can be switched on and off. Research is showing that along with what you consume, your thoughts, feelings, emotions, stress level, quality of sleep, and even your relationships influence the way your genes are expressed. It's as if your genetic code has light switches and you can turn some genes on and other genes off.

This growing field of study is quickly unraveling everything we thought we knew about how genes are expressed. It sheds light on how lifestyle behavior—our choices—influence gene expression generationally. How your parents, and even your grandparents, lived their lives influences how your genes are expressed; and how you live your life will affect your children's gene expression.

It might be your body, but your daily habits and lifestyle choices will influence the health of generations to come. What kind of genetic legacy do you want to leave your children, grandchildren, and your great-grandchildren? Even if you don't have children, have passed the childbearing years, or you don't plan to have more children, the example you set and the habits you teach to the children in your life is vital to the health of future generations.

A TOOLKiT FOR OPTiMAL HEALTH

~

MiND, BODY, & SPiRiT

All the knowledge in the world won't make a real difference in your life if you don't apply what you think you know or what you learn anew. This is true in all areas of your life. As an example, you may know what scripture says, but transformation happens as those principles are applied in your daily life. The same is true with health. You know what to do—eat better and exercise more—but transformation comes as you take action and make the necessary changes to affect the change you are seeking in your life.

Use the following pages as a toolkit. This toolkit is designed to bring awareness to a variety of factors that may be derailing your best efforts to be healthier. The information is offered as an instigator and a guide to a healthier, happier you—mind, body, and spirit! I hope you continue your research beyond the content included in these pages. Be curious. Ask questions.

This book is designed to help you create that transformational change. It can help you navigate the health and wellness information jungle and help you choose what steps you will take to improve your health.

Parenthetical numbers (1) are references. The references are organized by chapter at the end of this book.

Most chapters conclude with questions for you to assess your current lifestyle behaviors and what changes you will make to facilitate the transformation you desire in your overall wellness.

Live well, be well!

THERE'S TOO MUCH ON MY PLATE!

When you hear the word "nutrition" what do you think of first? Counting calories, eating healthy, vitamins, juicing, shakes, diet?

The food you put on your plate (or eat straight out of the bag, or refrigerator, standing at your kitchen counter, in the car, or hiding in the closet) plays a vital role in nutrition and the nourishment you receive, or don't receive. But before I talk more deeply about the food you eat and the role it plays in nutrition, let's talk about nutrition beyond the plate.

I hear it often: "I have too much on my plate!" Maybe you have said it? Typically, the plate referred to here is the plate of life. Often, busy people feel they have too many plates spinning at once because there is so much to do: work, build a business, family responsibilities—meals, laundry, shopping, school or work activities, volunteer in community or church ministries, etc.

Have you heard these food metaphor questions, "What feeds your soul?" "I bit off more than I can chew!" "That's food for thought." Or, one of my favorites: "I went to church today and I didn't get fed." (I'm not sure I understand how a person can be in the presence of God and not be "fed," but that's for another conversation.) My point is this: humans experience care and feeding far beyond the dinner plate. Optimal health, or wellbeing, includes physical, mental, and spiritual health. If that which fills you up and brings meaning in your life is out of balance, or non-existent, your health will suffer.

Your level of satisfaction, the joy you experience in your relationships, your spiritual life, and your work all play a role in your overall wellbeing.

Let me give you an example. Have you ever been so involved in a meaningful conversation, a work project, prayer, or outdoor activity and you lost track of time? What were you thinking about during those times? Were you thinking of food? Most likely not.

When you're actively engaged in activities that bring joy, life is enriched and nourished on a whole different level.

Humans hunger for joy, play, intimacy, love, a sense of peace, and even success. When you crave these things "beyond the plate" but stuff yourself with "food" to alleviate that hunger, you feed the wrong hunger. When this hunger goes unanswered, there can be a negative impact on the body and the mind and even on the spirit.

The food on your plate (proteins, carbohydrates, and fat) takes a back seat to the food beyond the plate when it comes to health and happiness. If you're not nourishing yourself—beyond the plate—with the activities and relationships which bring you joy, all the food in the world won't satisfy your "hunger." Food may nourish your body and taste incredible, but it doesn't bring you lasting joy. For example, eating chocolate may feel joyful at the moment but that type of joy doesn't last nor will it bring fulfillment or meaning.

Nourishment beyond the plate is at the core of creating a healthy lifestyle. You can eat the healthiest food on the planet, exercise every day, and drink plenty of water, but, if you have strife in a relationship, your job does more to deplete than fill you up, or you're lacking spiritual direction, you'll be stuck, and continue to struggle to meet your wellness goals. Make time to play. Make time for loved ones. Connect with your Creator on a deeper level. Do what you love to do every day.

What are you neglecting for the sake of time? In what ways do you use food to feed your deep need for nourishment beyond the plate? Take a few minutes to consider what feeds your soul. Are you starving for more of that in your life?

Reflect on your current lifestyle behavior:
1. How is your relationship with your spouse? Children? Colleagues? Friends?
2. Do you absolutely LOVE your job or career? If not, what would you LOVE to do?
3. Which spiritual practices do you routinely engage in? (Prayer, meditation, worship)
4. What brings meaning to your life?
5. How do you serve others?
6. What hobbies do you engage in? What ignites your creativity?

Transform your life:
1. What changes will you make to improve the quality of your life beyond the plate?
2. What will be the biggest challenge for you?
3. How will you overcome that challenge?

HAND OVER THE DONUT AND NO ONE GETS HURT!

Before you can embrace change it's essential to take a hard look at where you are—emotionally, physically, and mentally—so you know what needs to change for you. For example, if you want to change a compulsion to eat sugar, you must look at what drives that craving for sugar. Is it a physiological response? Is it emotional? What are you craving and why are you craving it? What triggers the craving? Keep in mind that a trigger may be a deficiency in your life beyond the plate. Is there something beyond the plate—your relationships, your vocation, your spiritual life—that's lacking in your life? Is there a void you're trying to fill with food?

Many people view cravings as weakness, but cravings could be messages meant to inform you of your body's physical and emotional needs. When you experience a craving, deconstruct it. Ask yourself, what your body wants or needs and why?

Here are a few more craving triggers to consider:
- Dehydration can manifest as hunger, so when you get a craving drink a full glass of water before you reach for food. Excess water can cause cravings as well, so be sure that your water intake is well-balanced. Most experts recommend that we drink half our body weight in ounces to stay well hydrated.
- Cravings may be a response to something you eat or drink (like sugar, highly processed junk food, sugary beverages) that spike your blood sugar triggering a craving for more, more, more.
- A lack of nutrients can trigger cravings. Inadequate mineral levels can produce salt cravings. Overall inadequate nutrition produces cravings for non-nutritional forms of energy, like caffeine and refined sugar. Junk food—or food void of any nutritional content—can leave a body craving more food, seeking adequate nutrition.
- A special childhood memory can lead to a craving for food that's attached to those special memories. What is the memory? Is it a hug, or time with a loved one that you're craving?
- When women experience menstruation, pregnancy, or menopause, fluctuating testosterone and estrogen levels may cause unique cravings.
- Sometimes a craving is caused by the consumption of caffeine, sugar, bread, cigarettes, etc.
- When you're sleep-deprived those hunger hormones and insulin signals are disrupted. Lack of sleep triggers brain reward pathways. Lack of sleep also reduces brain

function and our ability to make wise decisions. Studies show that when sleep deprived, people are more inclined to reach for junk food. Lack of sleep is linked to weight gain. Get your zzzz's! But not too many! Too much sleep can lead to weight gain as well. Know your body and your sleep needs to determine what is optimal for you. See the chapter Get Your Z's.
- Your own willpower may not be enough. The bacteria in your gut want and need sugar. They feed on it. They have a powerful will to survive.

These actions will help you navigate through a craving or decrease their occurrences:
- Stay hydrated.
- Exercise.
- Get sufficient quality sleep.
- Reduce stress levels.
- Call a coach, accountability partner, or friend to help you stay on track and root for you.
- Drink a cup of naturally caffeine-free tea. Yogi, Numi, Traditional Medicines, and Mighty Leaf have some great options.
- If all else fails, reach for nuts and some berries or a protein smoothie—something that won't spike your blood sugar.

The goal is to implement simple changes that become long-term habits. In any given moment you have a choice. Give yourself some grace if you make a decision that doesn't serve you. Begin noticing your thought patterns. If you KNOW that one piece of candy will lead to another, and another, and another piece of candy—decide if you want to go down that rabbit trail. Will that one piece of candy, donut, or pastry be a treat or a trick? Will it sabotage your health goals? Claim the 90/10 rule as you begin to make changes. Do the best you can 90 percent of the time and allow for special occasions 10 percent of the time. OR, start with 70/30 and work your way up.

As you move forward, remember to pay attention to your cravings and what triggers the cravings. Use a food journal to keep track. Awareness leads to the highest potential for changing how you respond to the craving triggers. Does eating sugar trigger the craving for more sugar and other highly processed foods? Is the craving due to an emotional trigger? Do you need more water, more exercise, or a chat with a friend? What action can you take to diminish the craving?

One of the things that helped me reduce and eventually remove sugar cravings was to eat more sweet vegetables: carrots, onions, beets, winter squash, sweet potatoes, turnips, parsnips, and rutabagas. Raw, roasted, added to soup, or made into a vegetable puree, these vegetables helped to reduce my cravings for sweet. You'll be amazed at how sweet, and delicious, a plain sweet potato without any toppings tastes when you give your taste buds and your body a break from sugar and artificial flavors.

Increase these foods and beverages in your diet (unless you have an allergy or sensitivity):
- Cruciferous vegetables (broccoli, cabbage, etc.)
- Berries

- Whole grains
- Humanely and pasture-raised animal protein
- Organic dairy products
- Pasture-raised organic eggs
- Wild caught fish
- Healthy oils (coconut, avocado, olive oil, grass-fed butter or ghee)
- Avocado
- Raw chocolate
- Raw nuts and seeds
- Chia seeds
- Organic caffeine-free tea
- Plain filtered water
- Infused filtered water

Reduce **these foods:**
- Chemicalized artificial food
- Processed foods
- Refined grains
- Conventional meats and dairy
- Caffeine (if you're sensitive)
- Soft drinks
- Alcohol
- Sugar
- Artificial sweeteners
- Trans fats

As you add healthier foods and beverages, your taste buds and even your cravings will change. You may even wake up one day craving a carrot stick or a green juice. It begins by consciously filling up on healthy (for you) food that feeds and fuels your body. You'll become less hungry for food with little to no nutritional value. When you choose healthier foods even when you don't "feel like it," soon your body will feel like it!

Reflect on your current lifestyle behavior:
1. What do you typically crave?
2. What do you think your body is trying to tell you?
3. How do you deal with cravings?

Transform your life:
1. What cravings do you wish to remove?
2. How do you plan to deal with cravings as you move forward?
3. What will be the biggest challenge for you?
4. How will you overcome that challenge?

GET OFF THE DiET ROLLER COASTER

Stop "dieting." I told you my history with dieting. I stayed frustrated! When on a diet, I'd diligently prepare and eat meals according to the meal plan for the duration of the diet and I would lose a few pounds—maybe. My husband, on the other hand, lost so much weight—eating the same meals I was—that he'd sneak candy bars to sustain his energy and stop his weight loss. When I went off the "diet," the weight I lost quickly returned—along with a few bonus pounds.

I had to stop thinking of a diet as something to go on and then off. Have you ever been on a diet and you found yourself saying, "I can't wait to go off this diet so I can eat bread again!"? Going on a diet implies you will eventually go off a diet. Instead of thinking of a diet as something you do temporarily, think of diet as your daily nutrient consumption.

You've probably heard about many of the most popular "diets" out there: Weight Watchers, Mediterranean, South Beach, Paleo, Whole30, Keto, Atkins, low-carb, high-carb, vegetarian diet, vegan diet—and so on. Have you ever had a friend lose a ton of weight doing a specific "diet" and when you tried it for yourself you ended up gaining weight, or gained back all the weight you originally lost? I know I have. Look at how many cookbooks, diet how-to books, and cleanse programs are on the market. Those books and programs wouldn't continue to sell if they were not helping somebody lose weight or get healthier. But they don't help all people. In case you haven't noticed, some diets just won't work for you. Your dietary needs may be connected to your blood type, your heritage, or even a medical condition. Your dietary "needs" are different from mine and may even be different from the dietary needs of your family.

Most diets remove (or restrict) food groups or restrict calories to an upper limit. The body needs fat, carbohydrates, and proteins to function properly. Contrary to popular opinion, sugar is not a food group. Food is much more than a calorie. A calorie is a unit of energy that fuels the body; we need calories. Yet, I think we do our bodies and our health a disservice when we count a simple refined carb calorie, a complex carb calorie, a protein calorie, and a fat calorie as equal.

One challenge for people thinking about a cleanse, or a diet, is the need to "give up" certain foods. Let's talk about the "giving up" part. You don't have to give up any particular food. You have total power to choose what to eat, or not to eat. Learn about the nutritional aspects of food, and beverages, and then decide what works best for you. Your decision might be based on how you feel after you eat certain foods. If you experience a rash, gas, bloating, or diarrhea, you know immediately that a particular food negatively impacts you and you should stop eating it. Part of the decision is discovering for yourself how a specific food impacts your body. The most effective "diet" is to remove inflammatory foods (see page 84). The best way to do that is to remove certain foods for a period of time—typically 14-28 days—then add them in one at a time and annotate what, if any, reaction you experience. Or, you may choose to remove a specific food based on informed knowledge about the effects that food may have on your body—long before you feel any effects via symptoms. By the time you experience symptoms, the damage is already taking place.

I hear many people say they want to be a healthier weight. They want relief from indigestion. They want an energy boost. They want to sleep better. They want. They want. They want. And they want coffee, sugar, bread, pasta, and other processed foods that excite the taste buds, give a temporary energy rush, or provide comfort. What do you want? I know you already know this, but I'll state the obvious; if you aren't as healthy as you want to be, you can't continue to eat the same foods that brought you to where you are right now AND expect to get the health results you want.

When it comes to food, wants (satisfying taste buds and cravings) don't always supply needs (food the body recognizes and uses for energy). For example, I may "want" a bowl of Cocoa Puffs. But that bowl of Cocoa Puffs will do little, or nothing at all, for my nutritional needs and may even cause harm over time. I want cheese, but I know it affects how I feel. You might want a piece of cake. I understand. Instead, of choosing what you consume by how things taste, try choosing by how you want to feel after you have eaten what you want to eat. Ask yourself, "How will I feel after I eat this? Will this create health, or sickness?"

Food can be complicated or, it can be simple. Here is the simple part. Most experts agree that eating fresh fruits and vegetables, unprocessed, pesticide-free, hormone-free, and chemical-free animal proteins will significantly improve the health of all people. The rest of it can be simple too. If you feel worse when you eat something, don't eat it. If you feel great when you eat certain foods, eat them. Be honest with yourself. Often people don't connect the pain in their joints with the food on the plate. Saying a particular type of food doesn't affect you doesn't make it so; it may be that you haven't experienced any symptoms, yet.

As you move forward, focus on what you want your health story to be. Diet is one aspect of a healthy lifestyle. Along with movement, spiritual practices, self-care, adequate sleep, stress management, and hydration, your diet plays a role in your overall wellbeing. How do you want to feel tomorrow, in 28 days, next year? What changes are you willing to make? See yourself at the end of one year and write down how you feel. What does your energy level look like? What have you accomplished towards transforming your life? Keep your focus on what you want your health outcome to be. Focus on all the good you will gain and all the excess weight and pain you'll release instead of being preoccupied with what you're giving up.

Reflect on your current lifestyle behavior:
1. How many "diets" have you been on? What worked? What didn't? Did you experience lasting results?
2. What do you want to change about your health story?
3. What are you holding on to that you need to release?
4. On a scale of 1-10, how willing are you to make changes in your diet and lifestyle?

Transform your life:
1. What changes will you make?
2. What will be the biggest challenge for you?
3. How will you overcome that challenge?

Wake the Health Up

WHAT'S FOOD GOT TO DO WiTH iT?

The body needs food to survive. Food supplies the fuel and nutrients that the body needs to function. This is a simplified, quick overview of why we NEED food. Food supplies:

- Proteins—in animal and plant sources build and repair muscles and break down into essential amino acids.
- Carbohydrates—are essential for the body to function correctly. Carbs are either simple or complex and are converted to glucose (sugar) to provide the body with the majority of the energy needed to operate. Complex carbs take longer to convert so sugar is released slowly into the bloodstream. Complex carbs are found in fruits, legumes, vegetables, nuts, whole-grains.
- Healthy fats—olive oil, avocado, nuts, seeds, coconut oil—help the body absorb some vitamins (A, K, E, D) and control cholesterol levels.
- Vitamins—we need 13 types of vitamins (A, C, D, E, K, and eight B vitamins)—to support digestion, growth, and nerve functions.
- Essential minerals—calcium, magnesium, sodium, sulfur, phosphorus, potassium, chloride, manganese, choline,

iron, iodine and copper are "essential." The body doesn't make them, we must get them from food or supplements. These minerals and others are used to perform many functions to build, grow, and maintain a healthy body.
- Antioxidants and other compounds that protect from inflammation and help regulate the immune system.
- Oh, and don't forget water. Water helps to flush out toxins and transport nutrients to our cells.

For the body to function optimally, it must receive proper nourishment.

This is a loosely based analogy. The body is like a car, let's say a muscle (Camaro, Mustang…) car. A muscle car is built to run on premium (high-octane) gas. If you choose to use regular (or low-octane) gas the car may lack power, the engine might knock, but the car will run—until it doesn't. When the proper fuel isn't used, over time the car will develop all sorts of internal problems not visible to the eye.

The same is true for the human body. Food is fuel. The body may function when given "regular" gas (nutrient poor food), but it doesn't function optimally. There may not be enough power (energy), the engine may knock (for a variety of reasons), and a person can still walk and talk. Until they can't. Remember, people don't wake up one day and suddenly have a disease or illness. The body has been "knocking" and trying to get attention—sometimes for decades. The body is divinely designed to run and recover when adequately nourished.

When the body is fed food created in nature, the body knows what to do with the food. That food supports good health unless we have an allergy or sensitivity to it. Food allergies or sensitivities happen for a variety of reasons—typically due to a compromised digestive system.

Have you, or someone you know, ever eaten a whole bag of chips? Not the individual bag…the big bag? Or the supersize Snicker bar that feeds four? A half-gallon of ice cream? Or maybe you ate half the half-gallon of ice cream. The movie of my life would prove that I have made some excessive choices in my lifetime. Have you ever overdosed on junk food?

Have you ever eaten three avocados? How about three or four apples? A whole bunch of grapes? A cup of almonds? An entire head of cabbage? No? Probably because your body can tell the difference between food and a food-like product. Real food is information and fuel for the body. Real food will satisfy hunger, supply nutrients, and fill you up.

Wake the Health Up

ON THE iNSiDE TRACT

About 2500 years ago, Hippocrates, the father of modern medicine stated, "All disease begins in the gut." Modern medicine is proving that to be true for modern lifestyle diseases. Health—good or bad— starts in the gut. (1) The gut, also known as the digestive system, gastrointestinal tract, GI tract, tummy, or belly is central to health.

According to the National Institute of Health (NIH), 60 - 70 million Americans suffer from digestive diseases. (2)

The NIH includes these conditions and diseases as digestive issues:
- Hernia
- Constipation
- Diverticular disease
- Gallstones
- Reflux
- Gastrointestinal infections
- Hemorrhoids
- Inflammatory Bowel Disease (IBD)
- Crohn's Disease

- Ulcerative Colitis
- Irritable Bowel Syndrome (IBS)
- Liver Disease
- Pancreatitis
- Peptic Ulcer Disease
- Viral Hepatitis (A, B, & C)

These are some symptoms linked to inflammation caused by a compromised digestive system:
- Abdominal pain
- Anxiety
- Appetite loss
- Bloating
- Brain fatigue
- Brittle nails
- Celiac disease
- Chemical sensitivities
- Constipation
- Chronic fatigue
- Depression
- Diarrhea
- Digestive problems
- Excessive gas
- Food sensitivities or allergies
- Gluten intolerance
- Joint pain
- Headaches
- Heartburn
- Insomnia
- Skin (rosacea/acne)

- Malnutrition
- Migraines
- Muscle cramps
- Muscle pain
- Mood swings
- Poor immunity
- Poor memory
- Shortness of breath
- Thyroid conditions
- Weight gain

Acute inflammation in the body can be a good thing. When inflammatory responses work correctly, inflammation is a form of protection. Inflammation, part of the immune system, is necessary to heal the body from an injury and defend against bacteria and viruses. On the surface of the body, signs of inflammation may include, swelling, pain, redness, and heat. When inflammation is chronic—ongoing—the constant inflammatory response, left untreated, stresses the immune system and leads to disease. Again, chronic inflammation is the root cause of most diseases. (3)

Learning how gut health can determine overall health triggered the "aha" I had around my own health problems and I wanted to learn more. So, I dug deeper into how the health of the gut impacts the health of the body and the mind. The study of the gut made me realize how intricately designed and connected the human body is. I could write volumes on the magnificent beauty of the gut and how it's connected to virtually every body system but for now I will give you a quick overview.

It's time to wake up and take notice of your gut. What if a healthier you could be as simple as caring for your digestive system? Nutrition, digestion, the immune system, cognitive health, and overall health and wellbeing are all connected and are critical to create and maintain a healthy gut. Have you heard the saying, "If mama ain't happy, nobody's happy"? Think of your gut as mama!

Let's take a look at how the gut functions and how it impacts virtually every aspect of your wellbeing. Amazingly, each section of the gastrointestinal tract plays a specialized role. Everything that comes into the body through ingesting food and liquids, absorption through the skin, and breathing, eventually makes its way through the digestive system for processing.

The gastrointestinal tract, the gut, is a very complex multi-functional organ system. It's about 25 to 30 feet long. That's one long tube!

Along with the gut, the digestive system includes the tongue, salivary glands, pancreas, liver, gallbladder, appendix, and microbiome. The role of the gastrointestinal tract is to be a transit system. It moves food through and out of the body. Along the way, nutrients are extracted and dispersed.

Do you know about 80-90 percent of the immune system, more than 100 million nerve cells and many neurotransmitters (such as serotonin, dopamine, GABA, epinephrine, and norepinephrine) are in the gut? (4) Upwards of 90 percent of serotonin is made in the gut. The gut and the brain communicate through the vagus nerve. The gut is considered a second brain.

Have you also heard this saying, "You are what you eat."? That's true. What you eat becomes part of your blood. However, healthy digestion is more than what you eat. You are what you absorb. You can eat the healthiest food and take the best supplements, but if your digestion is compromised, your body's ability to optimally use nutrients is greatly diminished. This can lead to troublesome symptoms or disease.

Digestion actually begins in the brain with a thought, a smell, or the sight of deliciousness. As you prepare your next meal—or walk by a bakery—notice what happens as you see food, smell food, or even think about food. I bet the thought of food probably has you salivating. That sends a message to receptors in your body to prepare for incoming food. And the digestive process begins. Saliva, full of enzymes, begins to form in the mouth. When we chew, the saliva mixes with the food and begins to break it down, and the stomach starts to churn out stomach acid, specifically hydrochloric acid (HCl), to aid in digesting our food.

HCl plays a role in the digestion of carbohydrates, fat, and protein, aids in the absorption and assimilation of vitamins and minerals and activates enzymes and hormones. The digestive system also defends the body against outside intruders. HCl protects the body by destroying ingested pathogens.

When HCl remains low, none of these activities happen, and a cascade of medical issues can follow. And those little invaders (ingested viruses, parasites, bacteria, etc.) can cause havoc in the body. (6)

When the HCl is compromised, the digestive process is compromised. Health is compromised! It's a domino effect. Is your HCl compromised?

> YOU ARE WHAT YOU INGEST, DIGEST, ABSORB, AND ASSIMILATE VIA YOUR MIND, BODY, AND SPIRIT.

Here are a few ways your body is telling you that your digestive system may not be working as well as you think it is:
- Adult acne
- Asthma
- Allergies
- Bad breath
- Bloating
- Burping
- Diarrhea
- Gas
- Gallstones
- Hair loss
- Heartburn

- Nausea with Supplements
- Undigested food in the stool
- Weak nails
- Vitamin and mineral deficiency

If you have one or more of these symptoms, it's possible your HCl is low. Each one of these symptoms can potentially lead to an illness. When HCl is insufficient, the bioavailability of vitamins and minerals is compromised and every function they perform in the body is affected. Iron, vitamin B-12, zinc, magnesium, copper, calcium, and selenium are a sampling of vitamins and minerals whose absorption is impaired. Consult your healthcare professional to test if your HCl is too low. Low HCl is much more common than too much HCl. It seems counter-intuitive, but many people suffering from heartburn, indigestion, reflux, or gastroesophageal reflux disease (GERD), have too little stomach acid (HCl) not too much. You need an acidic stomach for optimal digestion.

Several factors can play a role in reducing the production of HCl:
- Acid-reducing medication
- Age
- Alcohol
- Chronic stress
- Eating too fast or too much
- Environmental toxins
- H. pylori—a bacterial infection
- Lack of sleep

Leaky Gut—My what is leaking?

According to recent research, a leaky gut—or intestinal permeability—can be the cause of food allergies, low energy, joint pain, thyroid disease, autoimmune conditions, slow metabolism, etc., etc., etc.!

Chronic malabsorption can result from leaky gut and impact hormones, thyroid, adrenals, and virtually every system in your body. Now, a diagnosis may take up to 20 years. You don't wake up one day with a disease out of the blue. Your body gives clues—maybe in one of the symptoms listed above—sometimes for years!

What else can contribute to leaky gut? Here are a few culprits: poor diet, as in the standard American diet (SAD), poor digestion due to low hydrochloric acid (HCl) in the stomach, damaged microbiota, environmental toxins, toxic overload, and antibiotics.

How does the gut leak?

The intestinal wall is a barrier that keeps everything that enters the digestive tract from the outside world in isolation to protect the body. Microvilli line the wall of the small intestines and they absorb nutrients that have been broken down. The microvilli keep everything inside the intestinal lining and allow nutrients only meant to make their way out of the small intestine into the blood. Leaky gut happens when the tight junctions in the microvilli are damaged and toxins and large particles, not meant to pass through the intestinal wall, pass into the bloodstream. So, a leaky gut is a result of a weakened gut barrier that allows toxins and food particles that aren't fully digested to escape the gut into your bloodstream. Antibodies attack these particles seen as foreign invaders. Multiple diseases can develop or be exacerbated by a leaky gut. (6) Included are these autoimmune diseases:

- Type 1 diabetes
- Inflammatory bowel disease (IBD)
- Celiac disease
- Multiple sclerosis
- Lupus
- Autoimmune hepatitis

A molecule—zonulin—helps regulate the tight junctions in the intestinal wall. Gluten and dysbiosis in the microbiota have been connected with increased zonulin release. (7, 8). This results in the intestinal lining becoming excessively permeable (compromised), allowing large particles and zonulin to leak into the blood system. Do you have too much zonulin?

The good news is that a leaky gut isn't necessarily permanent. The gut can be restored. Do you have digestive issues? Work with a qualified health care professional who understands the role of digestion on overall health.

What can you do to better digest and absorb your food and support your digestive health? Here are three very basic habits that will give your digestion a boost:

1. Give thanks! Expressing gratitude is always a good thing and being mindful gives you time to stop and appreciate the food, how it was grown, who prepared it, and how it will nourish your body.
2. Breathe! Take three deep belly breaths. In today's hectic society, people live in fight or flight mode. In that state, all energy is directed to arms and legs so that we can get out of danger—fast! If you were fleeing from a lion, you wouldn't have time to stop and take three deep breaths! Taking time to breathe, or pray, signals the brain that you're not in danger and the body can spend energy on digestion (rest and digest). Support your digestive process—stop and breathe!
3. Remember when your mom said, "Chew your food"? Mom was right! Chewing your food 25-50 times (to the consistency of baby food) before swallowing aids in proper digestion. Slow down, enjoy your food. No more chomp, chomp, swallow! Eating fast, or gulping your food, won't support a healthy digestive system. If you gulp your food, you won't notice how much you're eating or notice when you're full. Chewing thoroughly gives your stomach a head start in the digestion process. Chew, chew, chew. Give that saliva a chance to work on breaking down the food.

Breathing and chewing may seem far too easy for a solution, but these are built-in mechanisms designed to aid the digestive process. Give it a go!

Here are a few more behaviors that help improve HCl, overall digestion, and gut health:
1. Use probiotics and prebiotics to restore gut health.
2. Drink up—between meals! Water is vital to every function in the body—starting with digestion. Reduce the amount you drink with meals to prevent diluting the HCl.
3. Learn how to reduce or manage the stress. Engage in exercise, meditation, breathing exercises, see a professional therapist.
4. Eat a variety of leafy green vegetables—if you tolerate them. Tolerate is different from liking them. Give greens a chance.
5. Include chia seeds, raw hemp, pumpkin, sunflower seeds, and sea vegetables to boost zinc.
6. Consume 1 tablespoon of organic apple cider vinegar first thing in the morning or before meals.
7. Drink bone broth (from grass pastured beef). Check out the recipe for bone broth in the Resource Section.
8. Avoid fatty, fried, and processed foods.
9. Drink peppermint tea.
10. Avoid eating less than three hours before bedtime.
11. Use digestive enzyme supplements to stimulate the production of stomach acid.
12. Avoid over-the-counter antacids. They may provide temporary relief of symptoms, but they contribute to other long-term concerns. Confer with your healthcare professional.

Reflect on your current lifestyle behavior:
1. How do you currently eat your food? At a table? On the couch? Standing? In your car?
2. Do you chomp, chomp, swallow?
3. Do you savor the moment and enjoy the company?
4. Do you experience any of the symptoms connected with digestive issues? What are they?

Transform your life:
1. What changes will you make to improve the effectiveness of your digestive process?
2. What will be the biggest challenge for you?
3. How will you overcome that challenge?

CLEAN iT UP, CLEAR iT OUT.

When I deep clean my home, it gets so much worse before it gets better. It seems excess junk and dust balls hide everywhere. As I move from room to room cleaning up and cleaning out the garbage, the piles of trash, items to donate, items to repurpose—or throw away—seem to grow. When I give up on the cleanup process midstream, I'm left with piles all over my house. In frustration, a pile may be moved to a closet, a corner, or even to the garage. This leaves excess junk and dust balls lurking in the last few rooms of my house. I wish there were an automatic clean switch in our home. Flick a switch and the dust, dirt, excess, and trash would disappear—wouldn't that be amazing?

Guess what? Your body—your physical home—has mechanisms in place that do the clean up regularly. Imagine a little internal Pacman.

Detox is a popular word these days. Before you "do" a detox consider that your body has built-in detoxification pathways. Given half a chance, a healthy body will naturally detoxify itself.

The detox pathways include:
- The liver—you gotta give your liver some love! Among the hundreds of functions the liver performs in your body, everything you consume (food, drugs, alcohol, even what you put on your skin) or inhale, eventually makes its way to the liver. There it's filtered before making its way into the bloodstream. The liver also converts fat-soluble toxins, making them water soluble so they can be excreted from the body.
- The colon—among several other functions, it flushes toxins from the body. When you're constipated, and waste sits in the colon, toxins can be reabsorbed into the bloodstream. If you're not pooping at least once a day—you're constipated.
- The kidneys—filter the blood and rid the body of toxins through urine via the urinary tract.

The body also detoxifies through the skin, lungs, and the lymphatic system. The lymphatic system includes lymph nodes, tonsils, adenoids, spleen, thymus and bone marrow. The lymphatic system is one of two major circulation systems in the body. Its role is to support the immune system. It removes and destroys waste, debris, pathogens, and toxins. It filters and transports lymph, containing white blood cells through the body. The heart pumps the circulatory system. The lymphatic system has no such pump. The only way to move the lymph is through an upward movement of the muscles and joints. If we don't move, all that sludge sits around potentially causing disease. Water helps keep that sludge moving as well. If you're dehydrated, the movement of the sludge slows down. The lymphatic system will back up and be unable to help excrete toxins, chemicals, and damaged cells.

Recently, attention has been given to autophagy, one method of detoxification in the body. (1) Autophagy is a biological process to detoxify, repair, and regenerate cells. It's one way the body clears out the trash—the excess debris caused by the natural metabolic processes created by living and by toxins we're exposed to. There is evidence that intermittent fasting, exercise, and sufficient sleep aid in efficient autophagy. (2)

Another way the digestive system takes out the trash is the migrating motor complex (MMC). MMC is a series of wave-like contractions in the stomach and small intestine that push out bacteria and residual food particles. MMC happens every 90-120 minutes. The process takes about two hours and occurs during a time of fasting. Eating interrupts this process. (3) The next time your tummy is growling, it's likely the MMC at work. You want this process to occur! Resist the temptation to reach for food.

For years I followed the recommendation to eat every three to four hours—five times a day. Three meals and two snacks. That eating schedule may still be beneficial for some people. But, it appears intermittent fasting (and sleep) is necessary for autophagy and the migrating motor complex to work optimally. There are a variety of methods for intermittent fasting. One is the 16/8 method. Identify an "eating window" of 8 hours and a "fasting window" of 16 hours that works for you. For example, eat your last meal at 7pm and eat your first meal —break the fast—the next day at 11am. If a 16/8 window seems overwhelming for you, start with a 12/12 window. Allow for sleep during your fasting period.

The best way to detox is to let your body do what it's designed to do. Remove inflammatory foods. When we feed ourselves well, the body begins to "clean house," clear out the toxins, and naturally detox and repair itself.

Inflammatory foods include:
- Gluten
- Dairy
- Sugar
- Refined carbohydrates
- Trans Fats
- Excess Omega 6 Fatty Acids

The best way to know what foods affect you is to do an elimination food plan. The premise behind this plan is two-fold. First, when inflammatory foods are removed from the diet, a compromised detoxification system can begin to recover as inflammation is reduced in the body. Second, foods that may be harmful to your health are identified. This plan removes the most common food allergens or problematic foods for a period of time—often 14-28 days—then reintroduces foods one at a time. Physical reactions are observed and annotated to identify problematic foods. Work with a healthcare professional to understand the benefits and side effects of a detox or elimination diet.

The first time I went on an elimination diet no one warned me about the withdrawal symptoms—detox symptoms—I would experience. When dairy, alcohol, gluten, sugar, corn, soy, junk food, etc. are removed, either one at a time, or all at once, it's likely that you'll experience one or more uncomfortable symptoms. Depending on the food and beverages you remove (and how many you remove at a time) you may experience symptoms for the first 3 days and possibly up to 14 days.

One or more of these detox symptoms may affect you:
- Headache
- Dizziness
- Fatigue
- Mood swings
- Irritability
- Nausea
- Food cravings
- Flu-like symptoms
- Brain fog

Don't let these temporary symptoms derail your long-term health goals. Remember, these reactions are temporary. If you do experience any detox symptoms, don't become discouraged. Hang in there and persevere. In a few short weeks you'll have more energy, fewer aches and pains, have fewer digestive issues, and have a stronger immune system. It will be worth it! You're worth it!

Help your body detoxify:
- Eat anti-inflammatory foods. Whole foods (organic when possible) close to their natural state to reduce pesticide and chemical residue. Include 3-4 servings of fresh veggies in a variety of colors (thoroughly washed).
- Move your body. See the chapter Move It, Move It, Move It for the benefits of exercise.
- Get a massage to aid the flow of lymph throughout the body.
- Use an infrared sauna. An infrared sauna aids in moving toxins out of the body.
- Keep your bowels moving. Don't start a detox program if you're constipated. If you have fewer than one bowel movement a day—you're constipated. The toxins you want to flush will have nowhere to go if your bowels aren't moving. Magnesium will help move things along.
- Breathe deeply from the diaphragm.
- Drink water, water, water. Drink plenty of filtered water— 64 ounces or 1/2 your body weight in ounces—to flush out toxins and keep lymph moving.
- Drink lemon water first thing each morning. Combine juice of 1/2 to a whole lemon with 8-12 ounces of warm to hot water.
- Add a 1/4 teaspoon of high-quality sea salt to 4 ounces warm water—drink up. Chase it with 8 ounces of room temperature water. My friend, and nutritionist—Karen Langston—shared this tip with me when I was experiencing severe detox effects. It worked!
- Go for a walk.
- Call a friend.

Consume these foods to help remove toxins from your body:
- Garlic
- Onions
- Carrots
- Broccoli
- Cabbage
- Kale
- Cilantro
- Blueberries
- Strawberries

Reflect on your current lifestyle behavior:
1. Have you ever eliminated a specific food from your diet for an extended period of time? What was your experience like?
2. Did you add that food back into your diet? How did you feel?

Transform your life:
1. Which actions will you implement to help your body naturally detoxify?
2. What will be the biggest challenge for you?
3. How will you overcome that challenge?

Wake the Health Up

HONEY, WE HAVE COMPANY!

Have you heard? You have company. Or, are you the company? Your cells, along with trillions of microbes, reside in the human body. Where did all these bacteria, fungi, viruses and other single-celled organisms come from? First of all, these microbes that live on your skin, in your mouth, in your nose—well, just about everywhere on your body—as a whole, are known as your microbiota. All of the genes that make up the microbiota are known as the microbiome. It sounds like a science fiction movie! Before you get disgusted, these little critters play a crucial role. They make enzymes that help in digestion, produce hormones, help to synthesize vitamins, AND clean up the toxins in your body. You may want to get to know these bacteria and the role they play in your health. Surprise! They even impact the way you think.

You may want to make friends with them—since they outnumber you ten to one. There are roughly 100 trillion microbes that you play host to. That's ten times more microbial genes than human genes in your body! (1, 2) The microbiome is actually considered an organ with "distinct metabolic and immune activity." (2)

The Human Microbiome Project (3) launched in 2007. It's a research initiative to "improve understanding of the microbial flora involved in health and disease." (4, 5)

It seems there are new discoveries about the microbiome every day. The science is still early, but it's fascinating. The science geek hiding within me is intrigued by all the new discoveries. When I learned how vital these little critters that dwell with me are to virtually every aspect of my health and wellbeing, I began to appreciate them. Holy Cow! It's more critical than ever to give your gut some love and make sure it's healthy! These microbes influence digestion and health.

There are "good" critters and "bad" critters, and when they live in balance, life is pretty good. In a healthy individual with a healthy microbiome, healthy bacteria and pathogenic bacteria do coexist. Although vitally important, the gut flora can get out of whack and create dysbiosis in the gut—which means your gut microbiota is out of balance. And that leads to all kinds of issues—even a leaky gut. Leaky Gut? Sounds scary? It is. Your gut can become "leaky" when its permeability is altered.

What can impact your microbiome? The microbiome is influenced by diet and lifestyle, (7) including:

- The health of your biological mother when you were conceived.
- Your birth—was it cesarean or vaginal?
- Were you breastfed or bottle-fed formula?
- Were you ever treated with antibiotic drugs? Yes, "ever."

- Do you consume refined highly processed foods?
- Have you been exposed to pesticides and herbicides?
- Do you experience chronic stress?

Obesity, alcohol, artificial chemicals, artificial sweeteners (8), infections, and some medications have a negative impact on your microbiota which can lead to opportunistic beneficial bacteria shifting into a pathogenic state.

The unnecessary and overuse of antimicrobial or antibacterial agents (9, 10) found in cleaning products, toothpaste, lotions, soaps, shampoos, clothing, and toys also damage the gut and your microbiome by altering the balance of bacteria.

The original purpose of antibacterial soaps was to protect at-risk hospital patients. Back in 2001, there were 700 household products with antibacterial agents on the market, up from 25 (or so) in the mid-1990's even though the benefit, or the safety, was being questioned. (11)

Antibacterial and antimicrobial agents play a role in the growth of resistant bacteria. Certain active ingredients were recently banned from use in over-the-counter antibacterial products because it was determined (after being in use for decades) the ingredients didn't demonstrate long-term safety. Of particular concern was triclosan, used in liquid soaps, and triclocarban, used in bar soaps, which posed possible health risks, such as development of resistant bacteria and hormonal effects. (12)

Avoid antibacterial soaps—wash your hands with soap and water. Good old-fashioned soap and water is proving the most effective in preventing the spread of germs. In a pinch, if soap and water aren't available, use a natural hand sanitizer to avoid triclosan and formaldehyde. Although not as effective as soap and water, use an alcohol-based hand sanitizer that has at least 60% alcohol. (12)

I used to keep a bottle of hand sanitizer with me at all times. I was a germaphobe. I had to protect myself from all the germs lurking on anything and everything I might touch—and I took it seriously. I definitely gave myself a squirt before touching any food. I didn't want any critters hitch-hiking a ride and making me sick. I have learned to appreciate these little microbes that dwell with me and discovered how vital they can be to my overall health and wellbeing. I'm now a recovering germaphobe.

Take care of your gut bacteria and they'll take care of you!

Reflect on your current lifestyle behavior:
1. Have you been treated with antibiotic drugs?
2. Do you consume highly processed foods on a regular basis?
3. In what ways are you exposed to pesticides and herbicides?
4. Do you use antibacterial or antimicrobial products? Which ones?

Transform your life:
1. What will you do to reduce your exposure to pesticides and herbicides?
2. How will you reduce your exposure to antibacterial or antimicrobial products?
3. What will be the biggest challenge for you?
4. How will you overcome that challenge?

Wake the Health Up

ABOUT ANTiBiOTiCS...

There are times when antibiotics are necessary and even life-saving. Antibiotics are useful for bacterial infections such as pneumonia, urinary tract infections, strep throat, and before surgery for patients at risk for developing infections. Antibiotics can't combat viral infections like colds, flu, sore throat, etc. One-third of all antibiotic prescriptions are deemed unnecessary. That's about 47 million prescriptions a year. (1)

Have you ever been sick with cold or flu symptoms, finally went to the doctor, got a prescription for an antibiotic, took the medication, and in a couple days started to feel better? I have. As I look back, it's most likely because the cold, or flu, had run its course.

A few years ago, I visited quick-care for large circle-like welts covering my body. When I asked the physician on duty what it was, he replied, "I don't know." I asked, "Could it be an allergic reaction?" He snapped at me, "I said I don't know!" Yet, he gave me a prescription for an antibiotic—just in case. I didn't fill the prescription.

Antibiotics aren't a cure-all. Taking an antibiotic unnecessarily won't alleviate the ailment, nor will it cause overt harm. It will harm your microbiome and cause a cascade of consequences within the body and potentially contribute to antibiotic resistance.

Antibiotic resistance is on the rise. There are some "super" bugs which include Clostridium difficile—C. diff—that are difficult, or nearly impossible, to treat because they're very resistant to even the most potent antibiotics. Bacteria are smart! Antibiotic resistance occurs because bacteria evolve and develop the ability to resist the antibiotics. More than 2 million people get infected with a strain of antibiotic-resistant bacteria every year, resulting in 23,000 deaths.

The CDC has created Be Antibiotics Aware (2) to promote responsible antibiotic use and to combat antibiotic resistance.

...and Probiotics

An antibiotic is anti-life. A probiotic is pro-life. About 125 years ago, the benefits of some bacteria strains—probiotics—were identified. Actually, the connection was made that bacteria could cause sickness or make one healthier—depending on the type of bacteria.

Probiotic and prebiotic use has become more prevalent in recent years, possibly due to the growing evidence that connects gut dysbiosis to so many illnesses. The microbiome can be damaged, and the diversity of the microbiome diminished, by modern lifestyle, antibiotics, and environmental toxins.

Modern medicine is proving the beneficial effects of consuming probiotics and fermented foods: improving intestinal tract health, enhancing the immune system, synthesizing and enhancing the bioavailability of nutrients. (3)

Studies are also showing that prebiotic, probiotic, and fermented foods can increase the diversity of the gut microbiome, thereby improving the functions performed by the helpful critters. (4)

As with any supplement, choosing the right probiotic for you can be confusing. Use a brand you trust. Probiotics are sold in supplement form, added to beverages, and added to food.

Probiotic bacteria are diverse. They even have names—well, they are categorized genus, species, and strain. Lactobacillus and Bifidobacterium are common probiotic bacteria found in supplements. Probiotic "names" can be confusing. This is how you identify a probiotic category: Lactobacillus (is the genus), rhamnosus (is the species), and LGG (is the strain). Research the genus, species, and the strain you are considering. Strains do specific things in the body.

Another thing to consider is how many colony forming units (CFUs) do you really need? More CFUs isn't always better. On packaging, CFUs indicate how many *live* bacteria you get in each dose. Some packaging reads, "at time of manufacture."

You want to know how many CFUs you get prior to the expiration date.

Fermented foods are a good way to populate your gut with healthy bacteria. Human beings have been eating fermented foods for thousands of years—if not longer. The bacteria in fermented foods helps to break down the food, making it more easily digestible, and increases the available nutrient levels of the food.

Choose non-pasteurized foods to gain the benefit of these common fermented foods:
- Kombucha (a fermented drink)
- Pickles
- Sauerkraut
- Kimchi
- Kiefer
- Pickled vegetables
- Raw apple cider vinegar
- Greek yogurt

Pasteurized dairy and foods are stripped of live bacteria. Sauerkraut is an especially helpful food because it contains beneficial bacteria and a prebiotic source of fiber for the bacteria to feed on.

Note: Prebiotics are not bacteria. They are non-digestible fibers that feed or stimulate probiotic bacteria—they get hungry too!

Prebiotic foods include:
- Asparagus
- Bananas
- Berries
- Dandelion greens
- Jerusalem artichokes
- Chicory Root
- Garlic
- Leeks
- Onions
- Raw unpasteurized sauerkraut

Keeping your gut bacteria balanced is important for many aspects of health so make sure you eat plenty of prebiotic and probiotic foods to keep your gut bacteria—the good and the bad—in balance. Give your gut flora some love.

If you currently experience severe gut dysbiosis, or other digestive issues, consult with a healthcare professional before adding (or increasing) probiotics, prebiotics, or fermented foods.

Wake the Health Up

MOVE iT, MOVE iT, MOVE iT!

When I understood *how* food works in the body, it was easier for me to make the necessary changes. Likewise, learning *how* physical activity benefits the body made deciding to *move it* much more desirable for me!

Just as no one diet will work for everyone, no one way to exercise will work for everyone. Some people will do better with a gentler, kinder form of exercise like yoga or walking. Others will thrive on vigorous exercise. For some, their body craves exercise, for others exercise is viewed as a dreaded "have to"—something they avoid. How about you? Do you get excited when you get to exercise, or do you dread the thought of it?

There are health benefits when you eat well, and there are health benefits—beyond calories in, calories out—when you move your booty.

Physical activity has incredible health benefits. Without it, you may never reach your full mental and physical health potential. You can't exercise your way out of a bad diet. Likewise, no amount of kale or quinoa will eliminate the need for your body to move on a daily basis.

If you currently have a sedentary lifestyle and you get very little to no exercise, just start. And be consistent. Walk 5-10 minutes every day and gradually increase your activity to 15-30 minutes a day. If you live in a hot, cold, or rainy climate, skip the excuses and head to your local mall. If there are stairs in your home or office building start using them. You can even do laps around your kitchen.

Research shows any type of exercise benefits the body—*every* body. Find something you LOVE to do and do it. Experiment with a variety of movement.

- Take a dance, Pilates, yoga, or swim class.
- Go on a walk, go for a hike, get a walking machine, run.
- Ride a bike.
- Use resistance bands. Stretch!
- Get a personal trampoline—a rebounder. A gentle bounce will benefit the body.
- Buy a jump rope—remember how fun it was to jump rope as a child?
- Join a volleyball team, play tennis.
- Park further away.
- Take the stairs.
- Play chess (just checking to see if you were paying attention).

Consistent exercise was a missing piece for me on my health journey. My personal goal is to use my rebounder and get in 10,000 steps (or more) every day and to learn new ways to engage in fun physical activities. Exercise is no longer a chore, it is something I enjoy—and even crave.

Once you start moving, your body will begin to crave movement. Maybe it's because physical activity stimulates the release of neurotransmitters, endorphins, serotonin, and dopamine—the feel-good chemicals. Endorphins also help relieve pain and stress. So, physical activity can also promote happiness and even relax you.

Additional benefits of exercise include improved sleep and a strengthened immune system.

Here are a few other benefits of exercise:
- Helps control weight
- Aids in digestion
- Builds muscle and strengthens bones
- Improves sleep
- Improves balance, coordination, and flexibility
- Promotes heart health and liver health
- Enhances mood and reduces anxiety, stress, and the risk of depression
- Improves insulin sensitivity, reducing the risk for type 2 diabetes
- Improves brain function
- Improves lymphatic system function and keeps it flowing
- Strengthens the immune system

Think of all the physical activity we humans engaged in before the invention of modern conveniences that allow us to sit, sit, sit, all day. Movement is vital for overall health.

New research shows that sitting too much is hazardous to your health—even if you get routine exercise. Stop sitting around! Get up and move! (1)

Remember the lymphatic system? It's more than a detoxification pathway. The lymphatic system absorbs fats and fat-soluble vitamins and delivers them to cells. It also removes excess fluid and waste from the space between our cells. The best way to keep all that "stuff" moving to where it needs to go is by moving—specifically jumping.

A great way to move lymph is to use a rebounder (personal trampoline). Your feet don't even need to leave the surface of the rebounder for your body to benefit. It doesn't get easier than this! Are you ready to commit to move, it?

Reflect on your current lifestyle behavior:
1. How many hours do you sit every day?
2. What physical activity do you engage in now?
3. How often do you "move it"?
4. What is favorite physical activity?
5. Are you involved in a sport, or two?

Transform your life:
1. The place to start... is to start.
2. What type of movement will you increase, or incorporate in your daily schedule?
3. What activity have you always wanted to try? Give it a go. Do a 30-day trial.
4. What will be the biggest challenge for you?
5. How will you overcome that challenge?

---

i CAN DO ALL THiNGS THROUGH CHRiST WHO STRENGTHENS ME.
— PHiLiPPiANS 4:13

Wake the Health Up

GET YOUR Z'S
THE BODY iS UP TO SOMETHiNG GOOD!

Feeling run-down? Do you have difficulty staying focused? Are you cranky, irritable, angry, or sad for no apparent reason? It may be lack of sleep.

While most people acknowledge that eating healthfully and exercising are vital first steps to a healthy lifestyle, the importance of high-quality sleep is often ignored in our fast-paced society. Catching up on the weekends isn't the answer. One of the most critical actions you can do to improve the quality of your mind, body, and spirit, is get quality sleep—*consistently.*

Sleep is vital to your safety, productivity, and overall health. Just as the body needs proper food and exercise, it needs adequate time to rest, repair, recover, and reboot. Your body is doing necessary work while you're just lying there sleeping.

Without adequate restorative sleep the body can't do the necessary work its designed to do. Depriving your body of much-needed sleep causes undue stress on the body, weakens the immune system, disrupts how your hormones function, increases cravings for sugar and carbs, leaves you with diminished mental capacity and can even lead to serious health issues such as heart disease.

It can be a challenge to get quality sleep. Today, many burn the candle at both ends. Doing more at the expense of sleep may seem like a badge of honor, but you deceive yourself if you think sleep is a waste of time. Sleep isn't a luxury—it's a priority. Not just on the weekend—every night. If you've convinced yourself that sleep isn't as important as your to-do list, think again.

Adults over the age of 18, on average, need seven to nine hours of restorative sleep each night. Yet, 50-70 million Americans chronically suffer from a disorder of sleep and wakefulness. (1) Are you one of them?

How much sleep do you get every night? Your sleep needs are as individual as your food requirements. Depending on your daily schedule, you may get more or less sleep. The goal is to have your body enter restorative sleep. Because you think you can get by on four to six hours of sleep doesn't mean your body agrees. There are bodily functions that rely on you getting your zzzz's to work effectively.

When you get enough sleep, you'll be able to wake up without an alarm clock, feel rested, and be ready to take on the day without a coffee cup in sight.

Critical restorative activities take place in the body during sleep:
- Internal organs rest and recover allowing for tissue repair, muscle growth, and protein synthesis.
- Hormones are released that help regulate appetite control, stress, growth, metabolism, and other bodily functions.
- Memory consolidation occurs! This allows for the formation and storage of new memories. Sufficient sleep improves the ability to learn new information. (2)
- Autophagy is supported. See Clean It Up, Clear It Out for more details on this process.

Too busy to sleep? Consider these potential side-effects of sleep deprivation:
- You're more likely to gain weight. The hormone that signals satiety, leptin, is reduced when you're sleep deprived. Leptin plays a role in appetite control and metabolism. Reduced sleep equals reduced leptin. When leptin is suppressed, your appetite and cravings may increase. This is likely because lack of sleep increases ghrelin which stimulates appetite. Test this for yourself; the next time you pull an all-nighter pay attention to your eating patterns and cravings the next day. (1, 3)
- You're at higher risk for illness. When you don't get that essential sleep, your body is more susceptible to stress. Stress impacts your immune system and blood sugar levels which can contribute to increased risk of diabetes, cardiovascular disease, depression, anxiety, stroke, and infection. (1)

- You're at higher risk of injury or accidents. When you're mentally and physically exhausted you may make mistakes you usually wouldn't make.
- Your brain's ability to process new information and store memories is compromised. When your mind is sleep deprived overall mood, focus, and cognitive function is impaired.
- You're more likely to be cranky, irritable, anxious, sad, and angry. Yikes! Give yourself—and those around you—the benefit of sufficient, rejuvenating sleep!

Tips to maximize precious sleep time for optimal health benefits:
- Get sunshine first thing in the morning. Get sunlight on your skin (face, arms, and legs) a minimum of 15 minutes throughout the day. Avoid sunburn!
- Listen to soft music, read, reflect on your day, pray, or meditate before bedtime.
- Invest in comfortable bed and bedding.
- Sleep and awaken using your internal clock. If you must use an alarm, keep it more than five feet from your bed.
- If you think you must keep your cell phone in the bedroom, put it on airplane mode and keep it at least five feet from the bed.
- Turn overhead lights off and use table lamps or light candles 30-60 minutes before bedtime to signal your brain that it is time to prepare for rest.
- Turn the heat down as you get ready to sleep and try to keep your bedroom at a comfortably cool temperature. Keep your room dark.

- Late-night snacking before bed, especially junk food and sugary snacks, will keep you counting sheep into the early hours. Plan your last meal to be three to four hours before bed, so your body is ready to rest and repair at bedtime instead of spending energy on digesting.
- Skip the wine (or any other alcohol) before bedtime. It may seem as if it helps you go to sleep; however, alcohol will disrupt your circadian rhythm and interrupt sleep and other body systems. (4)
- Avoid, or reduce, your daily intake of caffeine, especially after noon. There is more information about caffeine and the role it may play in your overall wellness in the chapter Gimme Coffee!
- Turn off electronics one hour (or more) before bed. Watching TV and surfing the web right before bed leaves you overstimulated and restless. If you have kids, set a no-TV-before-bed rule and watch their positive daytime energy skyrocket. Falling asleep with the TV interferes with restorative sleep. Any electronic blue light or light-emitting electronic devices can disrupt the natural sleep-wake cycle or reduce the quality of sleep by suppressing or delaying the release of melatonin, a sleep hormone that helps to regulate your sleep-wake cycle. (5) Does the thought of a technology-free hour every night stress you out? Don't panic! Try it. If one hour seems impossible, begin with shutting down all electronics 15 minutes before bedtime for one week then expand the time by 15 minute increments until you reach one hour.
- Breathe. 4-4-4 Someone shared this breathing technique with me years ago, and I use it to still my mind as I fall

asleep. Start by focusing on your breathing. Slowly inhale to the count of four. Hold your breath to the count of four then exhale to the count of four. Repeat. Repeat. Repeat. Sleep. This breathing exercise calms the body and sends the signal that it's time to rest.
- Leave the worry behind. There are times we lose sleep because we worry. Worry won't change the outcome of anything—except leaving you stressed, more tired, and focused on what you don't want.

I'm a recovering worrier. I used to think that if I worried enough everything would be okay. That's likely because those things I worried about never came true, not because my worry ability had any power! I learned to focus more on the blessings in my life. There were times I had to search to find a blessing. But, the more I looked, the more blessings I found. I changed worry to prayer. I found that prayer does change things—often the thing changed was me and my ability to deal with the challenges in my life. Prayer is one way of acknowledging that we don't have the power to change those things we "worry" about, but God does have the power. Lift up your worries, challenges, concerns, the desires of your heart, and give thanks with a grateful heart. Then do your best to rest.

Consider this: Do any of these symptoms disrupt your sleep?
- Loud or frequent snoring (your own)?
- Breaks in breathing while asleep?
- Choking or gasping sounds?
- Daytime sleepiness or fatigue?

- Waking up tired?
- Insomnia?
- Morning headaches?
- Decreased sexual desire?
- Memory loss?
- Irritability?

These are common symptoms of sleep apnea. Sleep apnea has many adverse effects on the body. Sleep apnea and sleep deprivation are proving to be hazardous to your health. Please follow up with your healthcare professional to restore healthy sleep.

Reflect on your current lifestyle behavior:
1. How many hours of sleep do you usually get each night?
2. Do you sleep with your cell phone closer than five feet—or under your pillow?
3. Is the TV on while you sleep?
4. Do you wake up refreshed? Tired?
5. If you're not getting optimal sleep, what might be disrupting your sleep?

Transform your life:
Give your body the high-quality, healing sleep it needs and deserves. If the tips to maximize your sleep time seem overwhelming or flat-out impossible, start small! Take tiny steps. Turn electronics off 5, 10, or 15 minutes earlier and go to bed 5, 10, or 15 minutes earlier and work your way up.

1. Choose one or two changes you'll make to improve the quality and duration of your sleep.
2. What will be the biggest challenge for you?
3. How will you overcome that challenge?

> PEACE I LEAVE WITH YOU; MY PEACE I GIVE TO YOU. I DO NOT GIVE TO YOU AS THE WORLD GIVES. DO NOT LET YOUR HEARTS BE TROUBLED, AND DO NOT LET THEM BE AFRAID.
> – JOHN 14:27 (NRSV)

EAT CLEAN?

Eat clean? What does that actually mean? While it's good manners to wash up before dinner, eating clean—today—typically refers to how food is grown, manufactured, and prepared. When I think of clean food, I think of food planted, grown, harvested, raised, and farmed the way nature intended. In the scope of humanity, the concept of "eating clean," unprocessed, or even organic is a new phenomenon. One hundred years ago food didn't need to be labeled organic. It was organic. Food was food. Food has gotten very complicated lately.

Making the food scene more complicated is the introduction of genetically modified organisms (GMOs). GMOs are living organisms—plants or animals—artificially altered by genetic engineering in a laboratory with DNA from animals, bacteria, plants, or viruses. Selective breeding for desired traits—like drought resistance—is a different process.

There are strong opinions on either side of the GMO argument. Are they safe, or not? Some say the data isn't strong enough on either side to make an informed decision. Yet, there are enough people—including scientists—raising a red flag about the potential dangers of GMOs. It seems further scientific study is warranted to prove safety to the human body and the environment.

Will you sign up to be a guinea pig? You really don't have to sign up; you are likely an unknowing guinea pig already because GMOs are prevalent in the US food supply. Apples, alfalfa, canola, corn (field and sweet corn), cotton, papaya, potato, soybean, squash, and sugar beets are GMO crops currently grown and widely used in the United States. Several genetically modified crops are fed to conventionally raised livestock. So, it's likely that GMOs are present in beef, poultry, pork, and dairy products you consume. Additionally, GMO corn, canola, sugar beets, and soy are prevalent in the majority of processed foods unless it is labeled USDA organic.

I am curious. Why are efforts to pass laws requiring GMO products to be labeled repeatedly defeated at great expense by the companies that produce GMO products. If there is nothing wrong with GMO foods, why not label them?

I wonder if GMOs and the pesticides associated with them will follow the same path as other toxic chemicals; although studies revealed the potential danger many of these chemicals had on human, animal, and environmental health, it took decades to remove them from production and use in the marketplace.

I wonder about the safety of GMOs. I wonder even more about the safety of what is sprayed on GMOs. GMOs were originally created so that crops could withstand the application, or spraying, of pesticides used to kill weeds. Superweeds now exist and require application of more toxic poisons. (1)

Some GMO crops are even bred to produce their own insecticide—BT toxin bred into corn, for instance. When bugs eat the corn, their guts explode. This type of corn is bred with BT toxin *and* is modified to withstand the topical application of pesticides—particularly the herbicide glyphosate. Some studies have shown that BT toxin and glyphosate can be harmful to the guts of mammals. (2)

The jury may be out (or "hung") when it comes to GMOs, but the evidence is mounting against glyphosate. The World Health Organization and the State of California classify glyphosate as "a probable carcinogen." (3, 4)

A product identified as non-GMO does not necessarily mean the product is glyphosate-free.

Glyphosate is used on GMO crops and widely used on lawns as a weed killer. Glyphosate is also sprayed on about 70 conventional crops right before harvest to accelerate the drying process and help the crops dry evenly. (5)

This a short list of conventional crops doused with glyphosate right before harvest effectively leaving the glyphosate on the crop as it goes to processing and to market:
- Wheat
- Oats

- Barley
- Grapes
- Cherries
- Dry beans
- Lemons
- Grapefruit
- Green beans
- Walnuts
- Sunflowers
- Pecans
- Pistachio
- Oranges
- Avocados
- Rice
- Sorghum

Food should not be to this hard to figure out.

The best way to eat food planted, grown, harvested, raised, farmed, (etc.) the way nature intended it to grow, is to grow it yourself. The next best option is to buy organic food from a source you trust. Get to know your local farmers and how they grow crops and raise livestock.

Some advocate that organic isn't all that it's cracked up to be. Sure, there may be holes in the growing process of foods labeled organic, but foods labeled USDA Organic go through a certification process. GMOs are prohibited in all USDA Organic foods. To learn more about the organic label, visit www.ams.usda.gov/organic. (6, 7, 8, 9)

It is a costly process for an organic farm, and organic food, to be certified as organic and carry the USDA Organic seal. I'm okay with that. I think all food should have oversight and be proven safe for the environment and human consumption before it shows up on store shelves.

The best way to "eat clean" is to:
- Keep it whole. Stick to "real" whole foods. A whole food is one that occurs in nature and wasn't created in a manufacturing plant. For example, fresh fruits and vegetables, grass-fed and pastured meats, dairy, and poultry, whole sprouted grains, raw nuts, and seeds. Know the farmer—and the farming practices the farmer uses—who supplies your produce and animal products. Whole foods free of processed ingredients, harmful chemicals in pesticides (herbicides, fungicides, and insecticides), added hormones, and antibiotics will fill you up, nourish you, and fuel you. Cravings for junk food will slowly go away. You may even begin to crave an apple, or other pieces of fruit, and fresh greens—because that's what your body needs. As you remove the noise caused by sugar and other processed foods, you'll increasingly be able to listen to the needs of your body.
- Get cooking. When you prepare meals for yourself and your family, the nutritional value is likely to be higher than that in restaurant food. Often, restaurant food is processed and over-seasoned. Start by cooking one more meals each week than you currently cook. Keep it simple.

- Keep your blood sugar stable. When you eat sugar and highly processed foods your blood sugar will spike—then plummet—creating an energy crash. If this cycle continues, you will feel irritable, hungry, and tired. Eventually you will become insulin resistant. Cut back or remove refined sugar and simple carbohydrates. This includes table sugar, white flour, pasta, pastries, and many packaged foods.
- Eat balanced meals. Whether you're eating a snack, or a meal, eat a combination of protein, fat, and complex carbohydrates. This will create optimal blood sugar levels and ward off cravings and brain fog.

Being whole and organic, or vegan, or gluten-free or dairy-free, or soy-free—or anything free—doesn't necessarily make a food beneficial for YOU. You are unique! Please keep in mind that people need and react to certain foods differently. Whatever you're eating, be mindful of how you feel. As you free your body of processed foods, you will have a clearer understanding of what your body needs and what sends it into a tailspin. When you keep a food journal, it will be much easier to identify reactions that are food and beverage related. A journal will also help you stay on track to achieve and maintain your health goals.

Listen to your body, but ignore that voice inside you that whispers, or screams, "I worked hard today. I deserve this piece of candy." "I have been so good on my diet, I deserve a treat." Or, "This has been a tough week—I deserve a break, a treat, anything". In reality, you deserve to be healthy!

Reflect on your current lifestyle behavior:
1. What does "eat clean" mean to you?
2. How many genetically modified products do you consume?
3. Do you notice an energy crash shortly after eating sugary, or processed, foods?
4. As you reach for foods that don't support your wellness goals, what do you find yourself thinking?

Transform your life:
1. What behaviors will you change to improve the quality of foods and beverages in your diet? Pick one or two to start.
2. What will be the biggest challenge for you?
3. How will you overcome that challenge?

Wake the Health Up

LET'S GET COOKiNG! YOUR KiTCHEN—THE HEART OF THE HOME.

For my non-cooking friends out there… don't zone out on me yet! Hear me out. I know some of you love to cook, some of you cook out of necessity, and some of you make reservations at the nearest restaurant, or you head to the closest drive-thru. Maybe you like home-cooking, as long as someone else cooks it.

My goal isn't to convert you into a master chef. However, I do hope to impress upon you the value of purchasing and preparing your own food and gathering around a kitchen table to share it.

Here's why:

We call it junk food and yet as a nation we continue to eat it and feed it to our children. If the nutritional purpose of food is to feed our cells, what purpose does junk food serve? When we eat "junk," our bodies are still left looking for FOOD—for nutrients to nourish and fuel the body.

Then there is "fast food." How nutritious is that food that comes through a car window?

When I was a child, I loved those Golden Arches. And while raising our daughter, we considered a trip through the drive-thru a "treat." Again, we must define, even redefine, what it means to treat ourselves and those we love.

I could lay out a whole host of reasons why consumption of junk food and fast food is on the rise, but the basic truth is—it's convenient and millions of people continue to buy it.

Home-cooking is healthier for you. When you purchase the ingredients that go into a meal, you have control over the calories and the quality that ends up on your plate. By the way, do you know some restaurants add pancake batter to omelets to make them fluffier?

Fast food and restaurant meals have more calories than you might imagine. Although calories may not be the most significant indicator of a healthy food option, it will become easier to identify the number of calories in meals from a chain restaurant. As of May 2018, the FDA requires calorie information be included on menus of chain restaurants with more than 20 establishments. The requirement for calorie labeling also extends to vending machine owners and operators, with more than 20 vending machines, who must provide caloric information for packaged items in vending machines. (1)

Restaurants are also required to provide additional written nutritional information for menu items. This information includes total fat, calories from fat, saturated fat, trans fat, carbohydrates, dietary fiber, sugars, and protein. Be proactive and search out nutritional information before you arrive at a restaurant—or even before you choose a restaurant. Nutritional information and their philosophy about food is often available on a restaurant's website. That salad you want to order may be loaded with hidden sugars and other ingredients you may want to avoid.

Eating out used to be my favorite pastime and I still love a well-made meal at a great restaurant, especially when the meal is shared with family and friends. However, in the time it takes to drive to a restaurant, wait to be seated, wait for someone to cook the food, wait for the server, wait to pay the bill, and drive home, you could cook, eat, clean the kitchen, and have extra time in your day for your meaningful relationships. And it costs less too!

Eating "real" food starts in the home kitchen. When I was growing up, there was a plaque in mom's kitchen that read, "No matter where I serve my guests, it seems they like my kitchen best!" That holds true for me today. Friends and family always gravitate to my kitchen area. If you have kids, grandkids, friends, or family, kitchen time is bonding time. Encourage them to play in the kitchen with you. Make it a family creation. Teach your children to cook and develop their love for nourishing food by encouraging them to make their own food. Practice your way to improvement.

For me, nothing is as comforting as a home-cooked meal made with love. Especially if it includes playing games, watching a movie, or engaging in great conversation. Preparing nutritious food may undoubtedly benefit the body, but it can also nourish the soul when shared with friends and family.

One of the best ways to maintain your newfound appreciation for whole foods is to get in the kitchen and start experimenting. Don't be discouraged! The more you "play" with your food, the more adventurous you become. You may discover the joys of kitchen time. Even washing the dishes by hand can be therapeutic.

Many people believe that cooking is too time-consuming. Cooking can be time-consuming, but it doesn't have to be.

These tips will help to make the best use of your time in the kitchen:
1. Cook once, eat twice (or more). Prepare multiple servings of meat or poultry at a time. Once cool, dice, slice, or shred and then freeze in meal-sized portions. It's so easy to pull a pouch out of the freezer and add a few vegetables to make a stir-fry or casserole. A meal can be ready in 30 minutes, or less. Be creative! Toss the protein into a salad, make soup, tacos, or a hash.

This is what we do in our home:
- We buy a large portion of organic chicken thighs and bake them with a bit of salt and pepper. We dice, or slice, the thighs in 1 1/2 to 2 cup portions and freeze.
- We roast a whole chicken or a small turkey, remove the meat from the bone and divide into meal-sized portions and then use the carcass for bone broth. Sometimes I roast a chicken just so I can make bone broth! Check out the recipe for bone broth, and a few of my favorite dishes, in the resource chapter.
- We cook three or four pounds of grass-fed ground beef with onion and seasonings and freeze in meal-sized batches.

2. Hard boil and peel eggs. Eat them whole or add to a salad.
3. Cook a large batch of rice or quinoa each week.
4. Cube and roast sweet potatoes, or butternut squash. Use in salads, soups, or hash.
5. Sort, soak, and cook a pot of your favorite beans. This saves time and money!
6. Use small appliances and kitchen tools to make quick work of cooking. My favorites are a Vitamix (or high-speed blender) for making nut milk, soups, and salsas, an immersion blender, a food processor, and a microplane for grating garlic, ginger, and nutmeg.
7. Mason jars, or FoodSaver vacuum-sealed bags, are useful for storing meat, grains, and beans in meal-sized portions.

8. Use a slow cooker. Toss all ingredients in and go on with your day.
9. Use a pressure cooker—get it done fast!
10. Better yet, buy an appliance that multi-tasks as a slow cooker, pressure cooker, saucepan, rice cooker, etc.
11. Use a salad spinner. This is helpful in getting those leafy greens dry in a hurry.
12. Wash your hard fruits and vegetables when you come home from the store to remove dirt and surface pesticides. Even organic vegetables will have some natural pesticide residue. A recent study (2) was done on apples to observe the effectiveness of plain water, a Clorox bath, and a baking soda solution to remove surface pesticides. Baking soda was identified as the most effective way to remove surface pesticides from apples. (Don't use that bleach bath!) The deeper the pesticide penetrates the skin, the harder it is to remove the pesticide—with any solution. Here's what you do to remove pesticides from apples and other smooth-skinned produce: Mix together one ounce of baking soda to about 3 quarts of water and let the produce soak for 15 minutes. Rinse and dry.

> LET FOOD BE THY MEDICINE AND MEDICINE BE THY FOOD.
> — HIPPOCRATES

13. Wash leafy greens when you're ready to use them. (3) Place your greens in a salad spinner and cover with water.

Stir in a teaspoon of baking soda. Move the greens around in the water then rinse, drain, and spin lettuce and leafy greens until dry. If you thoroughly dry romaine lettuce, and other hearty greens, they'll last a day or two in the refrigerator.
14. Wait to wash fragile fruits like berries until you're ready to eat them. Rinse and pat dry.

Going Against the Grain

Grains include wheat, oats, rice, barley, corn, and rice. Grains became a staple about 10,000 short years ago, give or take a few years. So, grains are relatively new to the human diet. There are conflicting views on whether consuming grains is beneficial, or not. Some experts claim that humans should avoid grains—even whole grains—as the human digestive tract was not designed to digest grains.

Other experts extol the virtues of whole grains. Grains are an excellent source of nutrition, providing essential enzymes, iron, dietary fiber, vitamin E, and B-complex vitamins. The body absorbs whole grains more slowly than refined grains, so they provide sustained quality energy. Refined grains have been processed to remove the bran and germ along with dietary fiber, iron, and B vitamins. When it comes to grains—as with any food—listen to your body. Do grains fill you up and sustain your energy or do they cause discomfort during the digestive process? Experiment and discover what works for you. If grains bother you...don't eat them. Remove grains from your diet for two to three weeks and then add them back in to observe how your body reacts to grains.

Phytic acid is a natural substance found in grains, as well as seeds and nuts. Phytic acid can inhibit digestion. Phytic acid impairs the body's ability to absorb some minerals (iron, zinc, and calcium) causing mineral deficiencies. Don't be too quick to remove plant seeds, nuts, legumes, and grains from your diet because they do have health benefits. Phytic acid does have some antioxidant properties. If nuts, beans, and seeds are part of your diet, soak them to reduce the phytic acid.

A great alternative to eating grains is to incorporate quinoa—pronounced "keen-wah." Quinoa is a seed. It's a complete plant-based protein and provides all nine essential amino acids. It also has a lower glycemic load and higher fiber than grains.

If grains are part of a healthy eating plan for you, this is the best way to prepare them:

Typically, 1 cup of dry grain yields 2-4 servings. Cooked grains store well so make a double batch for use later in the week.

Step 1: Measure the grain, check for bugs or other unwanted items (like small rocks). If you want to increase the digestibility and reduce phytic acid, soak grains up to eight hours. Drain and rinse in cold water using a fine mesh strainer.

Step 2: Add the amount of liquid recommended for the amount of grain you're using and bring to a boil. Typically, 1 cup of brown rice, quinoa, millet, or buckwheat is cooked in 2 cups of liquid. Depending on how you'll use the grain (on its own, or as an ingredient in another dish), use filtered water, vegetable stock, or chicken stock. Hint: if you prefer a firmer grain, bring the liquid to a boil before adding the grain. This will prevent the grains from getting mushy.

Step 3: Once the liquid comes to a boil, reduce the heat, cover, and simmer for the recommended amount of time (see the package). Don't stir during the cooking time. Some grain cooking instructions will have you turn off the heat and leave the cover on for a designated amount of time.

Step 4: Eat and enjoy!

Use grains in a variety of recipes or enjoy them as a side dish. Remember to chew, chew, chew. Grains—and other softer foods—still need to be well chewed and bathed in enzyme-rich saliva.

What's the Big Deal about Gluten?

Man does not live by bread alone. These days it seems a growing number of people are unable to eat bread at all. Do you, or someone you know, have celiac disease or non-celiac gluten sensitivity? Is it just a fad to avoid gluten?

The best way to know if gluten (or any food for that matter) bothers you is to remove the suspect food from your diet for 28 days and then observe how your body reacts when you reintroduce it. If you remove more than one food at a time, add them back in one at a time, a day or two apart. I encourage my clients to keep a food journal for the 30 days and track what you eat and drink. Note how you feel after a meal. What cravings or aches and pains do you feel? Be mindful of any reactions when you remove a food and add it back in.

Do you think gluten doesn't affect you? Remember, gluten triggers zonulin release which contributes to intestinal permeability—leaky gut. Actually, it is the gliadin—one of the proteins in gluten—that activates zonulin. (4) You may not "feel" or "think" that gluten affects you, but it is affecting your gut.

Part of the healing process for my leaky gut included removing gluten, dairy, and grains from my diet. In support of the changes I made in my diet, my husband didn't eat gluten or grains at home. But if we were at a restaurant or someone's home, he would "splurge" and order a sandwich or burger. He was resistant to eliminating gluten. He didn't have a sensitivity—so he thought. He was a few pounds overweight, and when he ate bread, he didn't seem to have a reaction. Yet, he had recurring bouts of reflux and severe psoriasis.

As we both learned more about the effect of gluten on the body, my husband decided to stop eating gluten. He feels much better when he avoids gluten. The reflux has subsided, and the psoriasis is improving.

Gluten isn't a "splurge" type of food. If you are celiac or have non-celiac gluten sensitivity a little bit can have an effect on your body.

Here's the challenging part…gluten may affect you and you haven't recognized its effect—yet. Gluten seems to have a wide-reaching effect.

A randomized clinical trial showed that short-term exposure to gluten may cause depression in subjects with non-celiac gluten sensitivity. (5)

Other conditions and diseases associated with non-celiac gluten sensitivity include gastrointestinal symptoms such as constipation, diarrhea, gas, bloating, brain fog, fatigue, joint pain, along with several autoimmune disorders such as Hashimoto's thyroiditis, and psoriasis. (6)

A genetic predisposition, consumption of gluten, along with a trigger such as stress, trauma, or an infection, can lead to celiac disease—considered an autoimmune disease. Gluten will trigger the immune system to attack the small intestine. When someone has celiac disease, minute amounts of gluten can create an allergic response, that can severely damage the intestinal lining leading to malabsorption issues. Like so many other diseases the incidence of celiac disease is on the rise. (7)

Gluten is a protein found in barley, rye, and wheat (couscous, kamut, spelt, wheat berries, orzo, and wheat germ). By the way, gluten is present in many surprising products. This is one more reason why it is wise to read labels. When eating out, ask the server, or chef, which menu items are gluten-free.

In addition to bread and pasta, gluten can be present in:
- Salad dressings
- Beer
- Gravy and sauces
- Supplements
- Soups & Stews
- Soy sauce
- Seasoning & spices
- Medications
- Cosmetics

These grains don't have gluten in them:
- Amaranth
- Rice (all varieties)
- Teff
- Buckwheat (kasha)
- Cornmeal
- Millet
- Oats
- Quinoa (not a grain)

Planning to eat gluten-free (or you already do)? Don't run out and stock up on the many processed gluten-free products available today. Those products can be full of ingredients that will not promote health. (Read the labels!)

Instead, improve your immune system, reduce inflammation, slow down digestion, and help stabilize your blood sugar levels by eating a variety of phytonutrient-rich complex carbohydrates (vegetables, fruits, whole grains, nuts, seeds, and legumes). These foods will curb cravings for white bread, pasta, bagels, cereal, chips, and sugar.

Eat well, live well, be well!

Reflect on your current lifestyle behavior:
1. How often do you cook at home from scratch?
2. How open are you to trying new foods and flavors?
3. What is your favorite dish to prepare?
4. How much processed—or fast food—do you eat each week?

Transform your life:
1. What changes could make your favorite dish healthier?
2. What will be the biggest challenge for you?
3. How will you overcome that challenge?

Wake the Health Up

GO GREEN! RED, PURPLE, ORANGE AND YELLOW TOO!

Your body will love you for it.

Leafy green vegetables. Love them or hate them—they're one of the most life-giving foods we can consume. The best way to promote health and build a healthy body is to add more dark leafy greens to your plate. Dark leafy greens are high in vitamins A, C, E, and K, and minerals calcium, magnesium, iron, potassium, phosphorus, and zinc. And greens have many micronutrients, phytochemicals and tons of chlorophyll, fiber, and folic acid. The more veggies you eat, the fewer anti-nutrient foods you'll crave. Have you ever heard anyone say, "I ate one piece of broccoli and I couldn't stop myself. Before I knew it, I had eaten the whole head!"? Me neither. Real food will fill you up without creating that crazy desire to binge. Eating junk food leaves your body searching for nutrients.

Experiment with adding some of these greens to your diet. Make a salad using a variety of greens. Add sturdier greens (kale, Swiss chard, etc.) to soup or stew. Make a stir-fry. Pop the veggies in the oven; broccoli, broccolini, brussels sprouts, zucchini, fennel, asparagus, and cabbage are especially tasty when roasted.

Get creative. Experiment with these leafy greens:
- Arugula
- Asparagus
- Beet greens
- Broccoli
- Broccoli rabe
- Broccolini
- Bok choy
- Brussels sprouts
- Napa cabbage
- Celery
- Collard greens
- Endive
- Fennel
- Green cabbage
- Kale
- Mustard greens
- Microgreens (baby plants)
- Romaine
- Spinach
- Swiss chard
- Turnip Greens
- Watercress

Greens play a *vital role* in overall health and vitality. Saying you don't like greens and you don't want to eat them is like saying you're happy living with the debilitating symptoms that manifest with nutrient deficiencies. Figure out a way to add them into your diet.

Let's look at just one of the minerals available in leafy greens and its benefits to the body: magnesium. There are about three hundred biochemical reactions in the body that rely on magnesium.

Magnesium plays an integral (to critical) role in:
- Muscle and nerve function
- Thyroid function
- Healthy immune system
- Activating vitamin D
- Regulating blood glucose levels and insulin sensitivity
- Heart health
- Brain health
- Cell division and DNA repair
- Anxiety and stress (1)

Magnesium aids in the synthesis of cholesterol which is a vital component of many hormone functions. Magnesium promotes sleep, which is also critical for hormone production. The hormone DHEA and growth hormones surge during sleep. Studies link low levels of DHEA to chronic inflammation, reduced immune function, rheumatoid arthritis, complications in type 2 diabetics, increased risk for some cancers, and heart disease. So, low magnesium is associated with elevated levels of c-reactive protein, and diseases such as type 2 diabetes, metabolic syndrome, and hypertension. (2, 3)

Insufficient dietary intake, alcohol abuse, chronic diarrhea, or a lack of absorption can contribute to a deficiency of magnesium.

This is one mineral—and the tip of the iceberg concerning the impact of magnesium on the body. Remember, there are more than three *hundred* biochemical reactions that depend on magnesium.

Estimates are that more than 70-80% of Americans are deficient in magnesium! Measuring for deficiency through a blood test is unreliable because only 1% of the magnesium in the body circulates in the blood. The remaining magnesium is found in the cells of tissues and organs and in bones. (3)

Symptoms that may result from a magnesium deficiency:
- Loss of appetite
- High blood pressure
- Fatigue
- Weakness
- Numbness or tingling
- Muscle spasms and cramps
- Abnormal heart rhythms
- Constipation
- Migraine headaches
- Digestive issues

If you have any of these symptoms, increase your consumption of greens and see if you have an improvement. Health benefits increase almost immediately when the intake of vegetables and leafy greens are increased. For fun, make a note in your journal when you increase vegetables and leafy greens and monitor your physiological responses. Track any changes in your symptoms and health.

In addition to leafy greens and vegetables, add these other magnesium-rich foods to your diet:
- Nuts (almonds, Brazil, hazelnuts, cashew, walnuts)
- Seeds (sesame, pumpkin, flax)
- Salmon
- Legumes
- Avocado
- Banana
- Figs
- Dark chocolate
- Raw cacao
- Quinoa
- Brown rice
- Oats
- Tofu

Flavonoids, a phytonutrient typically found in green and red plants have many health benefits including a lower risk of death from cardiovascular disease. A study in the American Journal of Clinical Nutrition shows even small amounts of foods rich in flavonoids may be beneficial. (4) Flavonoids also fight against cancer. (5)

Red wine, berries, nuts, and dark chocolate are excellent sources for flavonoids. Phytonutrients found in plants, whole grains, nuts, beans, and tea have antioxidant and anti-inflammatory properties that can enhance immunity, cell signaling, DNA repair from damage caused by environmental toxins, among other health benefits.

Some experts advocate against beans and whole grains. Know your body. In any case, it appears that a wide variety of colorful vegetables and berries is beneficial.

Reflect on your current lifestyle behavior:
1. How many servings of leafy greens or colorful vegetables do you eat per day?
2. What are your favorites?
3. Which, if any, magnesium deficiency symptoms do you experience?

Transform your life:
1. Which vegetables or magnesium-rich foods will you increase or add to your diet?
2. What will the biggest challenge be for you?
3. How will you overcome that challenge?

A GRAiN OF SALT WiTH A SiDE OF iODiNE

After weeks of flu-like symptoms, my father was admitted to the hospital. The initial diagnosis was complications from *"low sodium"*. He had previous heart and circulatory issues and was advised to adopt a low-salt diet in the 1990's. My father was diligent with his salt consumption—for years! He didn't cook with salt, never salted the food on his plate, read package labels and he avoided salt at all costs. He never came home from that hospital stay.

The body actually needs salt—neither too much nor too little. You may have heard—too much salt isn't good for you. For years experts have said that excessive salt can elevate blood pressure, cause heart disease, or stroke. But recent studies indicate health risks only increase when more than 5000 mg (2.5 teaspoons) are consumed per day. (1) Did you know a low-salt diet can actually have adverse effects on the body? (2, 3, 4) Salt is one more area where "experts" and studies can leave one confused. (5)

So, how much salt should you consume a day? Current dietary guidelines recommend 2,300 mg of sodium a day, for most people. This is the equivalent of about one teaspoon (or six grams) of salt.

If you saw a pile of salt on the counter, you most likely wouldn't dig right in. However, consumption of most processed food floods your body with excess sodium. If you want to reduce salt in your diet start by cutting down on canned and packaged processed foods. Read the labels.

To heed the warning to avoid or limit sodium intake, many people have reduced table salt in their diet. As a result, iodine intake is also reduced. "Iodine Deficiency Disorders (IDD) are one of the biggest worldwide public health problems of today. Their effect is hidden and profoundly affects the quality of human life." (6)

There is a growing iodine deficiency in the United States, especially for women of childbearing years. Iodine, a trace element, is necessary for making thyroid hormones which control metabolism. Iodine also plays a vital role in neurodevelopment of a fetus. (7, 8)

If you replace table salt with sea salt—Redmond REAL Salt, Pink Himalayan, or Celtic Sea Salt for example—it's essential to get your iodine through other means. Iodine, a vital nutrient, helps regulate the thyroid, and supports healthy metabolism—it's needed by every tissue in your body.

Include these foods to ensure adequate iodine in the diet:
- Wild caught fish
- Lima beans
- Organic cranberries
- Cranberry juice
- Raw cheese
- Bananas
- Prunes
- Sea vegetables (seaweed, kelp)
- Dairy
- Eggs
- Strawberries
- Potatoes

Wake the Health Up

GiMME COFFEE!

For years, the craving for, the search for, and the enjoyment of coffee drove my daily routine. It was a challenge for me to pass up the green sign with the mermaid on it whenever, or wherever, she beckoned to me. The sign was almost like a magnet. I always scoped out the closest location when I traveled. Due to the chronic stress in my life and the impact it was having on my health, it was suggested that I reduce or even remove caffeine from my life. Yikes! It felt as if someone asked me to cut off my left arm. I quickly discovered how emotionally and physically attached I was to my coffee.

I was not alone in my obsession; for many, it continues. Just notice the lines at a drive-thru. In a time when everyone wants it NOW, I find it curious that so many wait in long lines for coffee.

I've heard coffee referred to as "a drug in a mug." Although socially acceptable, caffeine is a drug and a stimulant. The thought of eliminating coffee sends some people into panic mode. Before you panic, I'm not suggesting you give up your daily dose of caffeine. Be informed—then decide.

Coffee is one of those hot topics! There are advocates proclaiming benefits of consuming caffeine, and there are those that warn against consuming caffeine. There is evidence pointing to 300 mg of caffeine, equivalent to about two cups of coffee, as a safe level for most *adults*. Understand how coffee works in *your* body—then decide whether or not to include coffee in achieving your health goals. Before you choose to allow the babies, toddlers, children, and adolescents in your life to consume caffeine, educate yourself about its effects on younger human bodies. (1)

Do you know that caffeine is also found in tea, cocoa, chocolate, decaf coffee, some medications (PMS, headache, and pain relief), soda (even non-cola sodas), and energy drinks?

Caffeine consumption can impact your body for three to five hours. Here are a few pros and cons of consuming coffee/caffeine for you to consider as you make your decision:

Let's talk about the cons first...
- Coffee consumption can deplete essential nutrients like B vitamins. Coffee can also interfere with absorption of many essential nutrients, including:
    - calcium
    - magnesium
    - potassium
    - iron
    - B vitamins
    - Vitamin D
    - manganese

- zinc
- copper

- Caffeine's diuretic effect can flush water-soluble vitamins such as B vitamins right out of the body along with magnesium, potassium, sodium, and phosphate. (2) Iron is a key mineral used in the production of the neurotransmitters serotonin and dopamine. Vitamin B6 also plays a role in the production of serotonin and dopamine.
- Don't take your vitamins and minerals with coffee! Caffeine speeds up your system flushing out the nutrients before they're assimilated by the body.
- Caffeine consumption increases the risk of developing coronary artery disease, osteoporosis, gastritis, stillbirths, and iron deficiency anemia. (3)
- Caffeine equivalent to four cups of coffee may or may not raise your blood pressure. (4)
- If you have diabetes, caffeine found in 2 to 2 1/2 cups of coffee may impair insulin reaction and cause a rise in blood sugar levels. (5)
- Caffeine is a stimulant and can cause increased contractions of stomach muscles and may cause abdominal pain, diarrhea, and increased bowel movements.
- Caffeine increases stress hormones triggering stress conditions in the body. (6)

Okay, so that was the downside. Is there an upside?

Here are a few pros for coffee consumption:
- Even at a low dose, caffeine has been shown to stimulate alertness and help you perform a variety of cognitive tasks.
- Caffeine can help the body absorb some medications more quickly. *However,* caffeine can create adverse effects when combined with meds. Do your homework! Compare your medical issues, your medications, and consult with your healthcare professional. (7)
- Some studies suggest caffeine can lower the risk of developing type 2 diabetes. (8)
- Some people report an improved sense of well-being, happiness, energy, and sociability when drinking caffeine.
- There are high levels of antioxidants in coffee. Coffee's antioxidants can guard against oxidative damage in the body. Drinking coffee (or other forms of caffeine) may improve immune function and reduce the risk of some chronic diseases, including diabetes and liver disease. (9) Antioxidants are linked to providing certain health benefits, including protection against some cancers and heart disease.
- In some cases, a moderate amount of caffeine can be therapeutic for people with asthma—but it's not a replacement for medications.

Well, I hope that cleared things up for you! Is caffeine good for you or bad for you? It depends.

Where caffeine is concerned, you're the best judge of your body. If drinking coffee benefits your overall wellbeing then enjoy a cup or two per day—size does matter here. Moderation seems to be a factor. Consuming 300-400 mg of caffeine per day appears to be the "safe" limit for some people. Pay attention to what *your* body is saying to you. Just because you *want* coffee doesn't mean your body reacts well.

Another thing to consider when choosing coffee is the chemicals used in the growing, harvesting, and packaging process.

I admit, I still love coffee—organic coffee. I love the smell of freshly ground coffee beans. I love the taste of coffee. But once I started listening to my body, I discovered three to five cups a day wasn't in my best health interest. I still enjoy one cup of coffee in the morning. I mostly drink water or caffeine-free teas. The green mermaid sign has lost its power over me.

The best way to know how caffeine affects you is to remove it for 14 to 28 days and then add it back in to see how your body reacts. If you decide to remove or reduce caffeine in your diet, do so slowly if you want to alleviate headaches and other symptoms that may occur.

Possible symptoms with caffeine withdrawal:
- Headache
- Irritability (that last nerve)
- Brain fog
- Anxiety
- Flu-like symptoms
- Drowsiness

When I speak of coffee, I mean plain black coffee. If your cup of coffee includes four pumps of—anything, and double whip, and, and, and—that's another topic altogether. Your taste buds aren't the best judge of what nourishes your body. Coffee may or may not benefit your body. All the other additives are another story. You must ask yourself if you're attached to the coffee, the emotion of drinking coffee, or the sugar and the other components in the drink. By the way, if you frequent your local coffee shop, consider taking your own travel mug to avoid drinking a hot beverage out of the plastic lid, or remove it altogether.

By the way, if you're reaching for coffee to give yourself a morning jolt or an afternoon pick-me-up, reach for water first. Feelings of fatigue and tiredness may be a lack of water. Additionally, if you're using coffee as a boost to make up for lack of sleep, a recent study shows that after three days of compromised sleep, caffeine has little to no benefit. And besides—your body needs the sleep! (10)

Reflect on your current lifestyle behavior:
1. How much coffee, or caffeine, do you typically consume in a day?

    Answer these questions if you consume caffeine:
2. If you drink coffee (or tea), do you drink it black, or is it loaded with all the "extras?"
3. How do you feel before and after you consume caffeine?
    - Do you have more clarity?
    - Do you get the jitters?
    - Are you able to sleep through the night?
    - Do you have insomnia?
4. Have you investigated how caffeine interacts with your medication?
5. If you have a medical condition, have you researched if consumption of coffee is of benefit or harm?
6. Do you use coffee as a replacement for sleep?

Transform your life:
1. What, if any, changes do you need to make regarding consumption of caffeine?
2. How willing are you to make changes?
3. What will be the biggest challenge for you?
4. How will you overcome that challenge?

WHAT'S iN A LABEL?

People spend hours reading product reviews for phones, computers, games, toasters, cars, etc. How about you? How much time do you spend researching these purchases? Do you research the food you put in your body? Do you understand what the ingredients are that are listed on the label?

My health journey began in the late 1980's. I started to notice that certain foods caused health related issues for me. Most of those foods were linked to monosodium glutamate (MSG). I began my label reading saga by searching labels or menu items for MSG.

In the 1990's when nutrition labels became mandatory, I looked for fat and carbohydrates on labels. I was told by a doctor—and the media—that fat was unhealthy, so I removed *all* fat from my diet. But I didn't pay attention to the other ingredients on the product label. The product was being sold, so surely the product and the ingredients were safe! Then I added a search for any form of sugar on the label and chose foods void of sugar—but artificial forms of sugar were acceptable (then). The primary reason I drank diet soda was to reduce the calories in my diet.

I didn't understand the health risks of sugar—I was following the doctor's orders. It was decades later that I became curious about the possible impact artificial sweeteners (sugar substitutes) had on my body. Now it seems widely known that artificial sweetener use has potential health risks. The science is unclear concerning the safety of some of the chemicals used in these substitutes. This is one area that requires more study. One thing that is clear is the obesity epidemic continues to rise in spite of the widespread use of artificial sweeteners.

Instead of reducing blood sugar levels, sugar substitutes may trigger the reverse effect and raise sugar levels in the blood. (1) The science is still developing, but it may be that these products alter the microbiome—remember those 100 trillion critters—which impacts gut health and overall health.

Dump the Junk

Many processed foods and beverages on the market today are void of nutrients themselves, and they contain ingredients that can further deplete the body of vital nutrients necessary for optimal function. Most packaged foods include a long list of food-like substances that do more harm than good in the body—including trans fats.

In 2006 when I was preparing for a Toastmasters speech, my attention to label reading escalated. I found it interesting that although the dangers of partially hydrogenated oil (PHOs)—also referred to as trans fat—were suspected in the 1970's, and confirmed in the 1990's to cause cancer, they were still permitted in the food supply long after the danger was recognized. It doesn't seem as if any amount is safe, yet this chemically processed product has been allowed to lurk in our food source for years (2). Trans fats are created by adding extra hydrogen atoms to vegetable oil.

In 2006, labeling laws finally required identifying trans fat on the nutritional label. The front of the product packaging could declare the item was free of trans fat if it was less than 0.5 grams per serving. For me, free means free. But in the world of labeling trans fats "free" means less than 0.5 grams per serving. How is that free? Labeling was required, but despite known dangers, there was not a mandate to entirely remove trans fats from the food supply. Until recently. A ruling from the FDA in June 2015 reversed the decision regarding trans fats. They're no longer generally recognized as safe (GRAS). June 18, 2018 was the cut-off date for which manufacturers can't add partially hydrogenated oils to foods. That doesn't mean processed food will be free of PFOs right away. It may be early January 2021 before they're finally removed from the marketplace. (3, 4)

You'll find trans fats in many highly processed and packaged foods including snack foods, microwave popcorn, baked goods, cookies, donuts, crackers, frosting, ice cream, dairy products, margarine, and frozen breakfast products. Look for the nutritional chart and ingredient list on the product label and avoid any food made with partially hydrogenated oil. Don't rely on the catchy phrases or health claims on the front of a can, box, or bag—read the ingredients. Trans fats are also found in fast food so remember to ask to see the nutritional information if you're at a large chain restaurant.

Most foods will have some level of processing. When I speak of processed foods, I speak of highly processed and packaged foods. If you eat these foods, understand what ingredients comprise the product.

I applaud the removal of trans fat from the food supply, although I wonder why it took more than 40 years to make it so.

The Cost of Convenience

It seems we often hear inconclusive or conflicting evidence about the disease-causing effects of chemical additives.

One ingredient currently under scrutiny is brominated vegetable oil (BVO). It was added to popular sports drinks and other citrus flavored beverages as an emulsifier to prevent flavors from separating. Some companies have begun to remove BVO. Read the label.

Once, BVO was generally recognized as safe (GRAS). Brominated vegetable oil is under review by the FDA as a possible toxin. Pending further research, under interim status, the FDA allows BVO to be used as a food additive under certain conditions. This status has been in place since 1977. (5) Most GRAS ingredients are considered safe when consumed up to a specific quantity. Some experts continue to question the safety of BVO—especially when consumed in large amounts. (6)

BVO isn't in every beverage, but most soft drinks (also known as soda or pop) are laden with other chemicals, food-dyes, sugar or high-fructose corn syrup. One 12-ounce can (or bottle) of soda exceeds the recommended daily intake of sugar for an adult. A popular cola contains 39 grams of added sugars. Imagine the amount of sugar you, or your children, consume with a super-sized drink—or unlimited refills.

Chemical food additives, BHA and BHT, are also added to foods to prevent oil from becoming rancid and to extend the shelf life. BHA and BHT are found in many processed foods including cereals, snack foods, drink mixes, gum, and beer. The effects on the body are under scrutiny. Despite being antioxidants, BHT and BHA may cause harm. Although some animal studies are suspect, health effects on humans are unclear. The FDA says BHA is safe although data from the National Toxicology Program says it's likely a carcinogen—other researchers say not. (7)

Read labels and know what the ingredients used in products you consume are, what they are used for, and the potential effects on health.

I'm curious why foods are removed from the marketplace only after proved unsafe. Is it too much to expect foods to be proven safe before they are released on the market?

Labeling laws that prevent companies from making false claims also prevent making truthful claims. (8)

It can make a sane person crazy trying to sort out the politics of science. Even when a substance is identified as a carcinogen, it takes decades to be removed from the marketplace. We can't wait for the government to remove foods hazardous to our health!

Labeling laws have been in effect since the 1970's and became mandatory in 1990. Changes were made in May 2016 to the Nutritional Facts and Supplement Label found on all packaged foods. (9) Although the changes were to take effect July 26, 2018, the date has been adjusted to January 1, 2020 for companies with more than $10 million in annual food sales and January 1, 2021 for companies with less $10 million in sales. There are three significant changes on the new Nutrition Facts Label I want to bring to your attention:

1. Total Fat, Saturated Fat, and *Trans Fat* are still required on the label but "Calories from Fat" are no longer required in response to research showing the *type* fat is more important than the amount of fat.
2. "Servings per container" is now in a larger font size, and "Serving Size" is larger still, making it easier to determine portion size. Have you ever eaten a small bag of chips, or cookies, and noticed the nutritional facts weren't for the whole bag but for two or three servings? Who hasn't?
3. "Added sugars" is a new category. The label still lists Total Carbohydrates, Dietary Fiber, and Total Sugars, but now you can identify *Added Sugars*. Applesauce is an example. Sugar is naturally occurring in apples; however, some brands, or companies, add additional sweeteners

to applesauce. This change will shine a light on the hidden sugars in foods such as yogurt, flavored milk products, jam or jelly, juice, tomato products, and granola.

I now read labels on virtually everything that comes in a package. I actually read the ingredient label on cleaning supplies, skin and body products, and almost everything I buy. The more I pay attention to the ingredients on labels the more I wonder about the potential implications on health and on the environment (which ultimately does impact health!).

Just because a product says "all natural" doesn't necessarily make it so, or make it safe. I believe we consumers must be diligent and know what we're purchasing. I don't consider the ability to pronounce a word indicative of its safety. Have you heard this advice, "If you can't pronounce it, don't eat it"? It might seem like good advice unless you're talking about probiotic strains.... That's like saying, "If you don't understand it, it must not be true." It's true for some words. Piperonyl butoxide, a man-made pesticide, for instance. However, Lactobacillus (a probiotic) may be very beneficial. When it comes to unfamiliar words, look them up before you determine the benefit or detriment of using the product.

So where does that leave the average person trying to make the best decisions for their family within the finances allowed? Start by becoming an informed consumer. It's time, as consumers, to raise our expectations and to be choosy about what we purchase and consume.

The landscape in the food arena is ever-evolving. Be aware. Do your research. Be informed. Yes, it will take time when you first start. It's like learning any skill...repetition, repetition, repetition! You'll learn which ingredients you want to consume or avoid. You'll begin to trust certain brands. However, even with brands you trust, read labels when buying new products within the brand, or to be aware of changes in products you already use.

Don't sell your health to the lowest bidder or the product with the catchiest advertisement. Good marketing is good marketing. Good marketing doesn't make a product good for you.

Processed foods labeled vegan, vegetarian, gluten-free, sugar-free, low-fat are still processed and may not be the healthiest options. It cracks me up when foods that are naturally gluten-free are labeled gluten-free and the price is higher. Items with any specialty label are bound to be priced higher than "regular" food. One study (10) compared the cost of gluten-free and regular foods; gluten-free products were more expensive. This may be because of cross-contamination issues that cost the manufacturer more money to resolve.

Here's a thought:
Eat a wide variety of perishable food created and sustained by nature in reasonable quantities.

A quick note about "studies." They are a complex thing: Are they controlled, are they double-blind? Who paid for the study?

How many study subjects? When was the study done? Is it based on new science? New scientific evidence is rapidly developing, especially in the area of gut and brain health. I find it curious what the FDA allows in the food supply. The burden of proof seems to be on the consumer, or consumer advocates, to show a product is unsafe. Why isn't the safety of a product proven before its release into the food supply? Consider, for instance, how long it took to remove trans fat, once considered safe, and then recognized as harmful long before it was removed from the shelves—in fact, we're still waiting for that. Reading studies is beneficial. Again, it can make a head spin. Often the literature is laden with language only a scientist, biologist, or other type of "ologist" can understand. But I wonder, if the safety of an ingredient is in question, why would you want to subject your body to it? If there is a question about the safety of a consumable product, why is it not removed from the marketplace *until* proven safe?

Wake the Health Up

SPEAKiNG OF SUGAR

Before you say, "I could never give up sugar!" consider the following:

Sugar reduces the ability of white blood cells to destroy toxins, which leads to inflammation within 30 minutes after eating and lasts up to five hours. Inflammation is the root cause of most illness today. Inflammation compromises most immune functions and also causes hormone imbalances. Consuming sugar prevents healing and interferes with normal gut and hormone function. Sugar also plays a role in polycystic ovary syndrome (PCOS). (1). Still not enough to convince you to convince? Read on.

The body converts much of the food we consume into sugar—glucose—for use as energy. The body needs glucose for energy, but does it need the copious amounts of added sweetener that floods the average body?

Another form of sugar, fructose, is metabolized by the liver and much of it is stored as fat. You may be surprised by how many products have High Fructose Corn Syrup (also labeled as fructose, or fructose syrup) in them. Read your labels.

The average American consumes about 17 teaspoons of added sugar, in any form, every day. (2)

It's recommended that the sugar intake for women is limited to 6 teaspoons (24 grams) per day. At 16 calories per teaspoon, that is 96 calories. For men, the limit is 9 teaspoons (36 grams), or 144 calories. To put that in perspective, one can of cola has 39 grams of sugar. Sugar is a prevalent ingredient in the food chain and you must decide if and how you will consume it.

Do you know how much sugar you consume each day? Are you aware of how much sugar is added to the food you eat?

Here is a sampling of the various forms of sugar:
- Refined sugar
- Raw sugar
- Brown sugar
- Castor sugar
- Cane sugar
- Pure cane sugar
- Evaporated cane sugar
- Invert sugar
- Date sugar
- Sorghum syrup
- Coconut sugar
- Turbinado sugar
- Honey

- Molasses
- Maple syrup
- Agave nectar
- Beet sugar
- Carob syrup
- Corn syrup
- Rice syrup
- Brown rice syrup
- High-fructose corn syrup
- Fructose
- Crystalline fructose
- Glucose
- Lactose
- Maltose
- Sucrose
- Dextrose

Whatever form of sugar you consume, sugar is still sugar, and too much of even a whole-food option (honey, maple syrup, etc.) is still too much. The body breaks down refined sugar very quickly causing insulin and blood sugar levels to skyrocket. When blood sugar skyrockets, what happens next? Emotions take a dive! When I eat too much sugar, I become tired, sluggish, hungry and I feel like I ran into a brick wall. Thunk! So, I'd eat more sugary carbohydrate for energy. This set my body on a roller coaster ride that was going to end one way—insulin resistance.

When sugar consumption remains consistently high, the body begins to lose the ability to respond to sugar in the bloodstream, and the pancreas releases more and more insulin to compensate. This leads the body to become resistant to insulin. Left unchecked, this could lead to diabetes.

Have you ever seen someone eat a whole package of cookies or a big bag of chips and not feel full? How about a pan of fudge? A super-sized Snickers bar? An entire pint (or two) of ice cream? Your body will have to deal with the fallout of that sugar rush—but you may not feel full. Eating sugar increases sugar bingeing and creates a dependence (addiction) on sugar. (3)

Stop giving your taste buds control of your health.

Whole food vegetables, fruits, and dairy products have naturally occurring sugars but with those sugars come fiber and other beneficial compounds like phytonutrients. You aren't likely to binge on this type of food.

Have you seen anyone eat a whole bunch of grapes? How many bananas can you eat? Can you eat an entire bag of apples or oranges? Probably not. The fiber in fruit slows down the conversion of sugar. This allows time for the gut to expand and feel a sense of fullness making overeating unlikely.

Next time you're tired, need a pick-me-up, or, you're actually hungry, reach for a piece of fruit. Along with the naturally occurring sugar, the fruit brings along water, fiber, and various micronutrients that the body knows how to process.

Do you think artificial sweeteners are the answer? Not so fast!

Artificial sweeteners became popular in the 1960's. They have been hotly debated ever since. There are studies proclaiming their safety, and there are studies questioning their safety. Despite the use of artificial sweeteners, the obesity epidemic continues to rise. Artificial sweeteners may be calorie free, but they have no nourishing value, and they do affect health. And again, you're not likely to feel full.

A study shows that the consumption of artificial sweeteners interferes with healthy gut bacteria. (4)

Daily intake of diet soda and other artificially sweetened beverages (ASB) can contribute to weight gain, obesity, and metabolic syndrome and increases the risk of developing type 2 diabetes and cardiovascular events. (5, 6) One study cautions that artificial sweeteners are increasingly used in other foods and "whether such products have positive, negative or neutral effects on body weight or other metabolic outcomes is even less clear than for ASB." (7) Awareness and limiting overall sweetening of the diet is warranted, regardless of whether the sweetener provides energy directly or not (natural or artificial sweetener).

Artificial sweeteners desensitize the taste buds to sweetness and can alter the way food tastes. As you begin to eat fresh, whole, real foods your taste buds will start to change. The old craving for processed sweets will diminish and be satisfied with the natural sweetness found in fruit or one of the natural sweeteners listed above.

Reflect on your current lifestyle behavior:
1. Analyze how much sugar you consume each day. Are you surprised by how much sugar you actually consume?
2. How attached are you to sugar?
3. Do you use artificial sweeteners to sweeten food or beverages?
4. Do you consume diet soda, or over-sweetened coffee? If so, how much?

Transform your life:
1. What changes will you make to reduce your dependency on sugar, or artificial sweeteners?
2. What will be the biggest challenge for you?
3. How will you overcome that challenge?

OBESiTY...iT'S AN EPiDEMiC!

According to some estimates, obesity-related diseases cost between $147 and $210 BILLION a year. (1) Childhood obesity comes in at a mere $14 billion a year in medical costs. Holy moly!

Despite the fact the United States spends $66 billion a year in the weight loss market we're getting fatter, not thinner. (2)

In the 1980's less than 10% of the US population was considered obese. (3)

According to the US Center for Disease Control and Prevention, "Obesity-related conditions include heart disease, stroke, type 2 diabetes, and certain types of cancer, some of the leading causes of preventable death." (4) Recent data from the CDC states that *more than* 36.5 % of US adults are obese. (5) This recent, drastic rise in obesity startled me.

One in three! That's how many adults are considered obese! And nearly one in six kids and teens are obese according to the Centers for Disease Control and Prevention (CDC). The rates continue to rise.

So, I wonder, if obesity is linked to heart disease, stroke, type 2 diabetes, and some cancers, *what causes obesity*? All these illnesses can be linked to digestive issues, too much stress, lack of sleep—inflammation in the body. These are all linked to obesity as well. Is obesity simply one more symptom—or result—of the body not properly functioning due to inflammation?

Most experts can agree that obesity is on the rise, but that's where consensus seems to stop. A myriad of opinions from the CDC to your local nutritionist, physician, functional medicine practitioner, health coach, or your mama about how to reduce obesity abounds. It's overwhelming! Some conflicting opinions revolve around grains (even whole grains), removing all fat, limiting fat to low-fat or non-fat, increasing healthy fats, and restricting calorie intake vs. calories don't matter. The CDC recommends whole grain, fruits, vegetables, lean protein, low-fat or fat-free dairy products, and water to lose weight. That's exactly what I was eating as my body weight escalated.

It seems reasonable to assume the cause of obesity is as simple as calories in and calories used. Eating too much and moving too little. I think it's more complicated than that.

What about the state of food? Is it the condition of the food supply? Is food nutrient-rich, or has the soil been so depleted that the nutrient value of food isn't what it used to be? Is it a nature-made food? Is it made in a lab? Is it highly processed? Is it laden with chemicals and preservatives? Is it heavily sprayed with pesticides, fungicides, and herbicides?

Is the body receiving and utilizing the necessary nutrients—or does it go in search of more food to look for nutrients? What about lifestyle? Is sleep deprivation or chronic stress part of the equation? Is exercise a daily routine? Or is the rise in obesity a result of all—or a combination—of the above?

What if the answer to reducing the rise of obesity is reducing inflammation? We must reverse the rising obesity epidemic—and soon!

Did you know that someone can be skinny on the outside and fat on the inside?

According to Dr. Robert Lustig, USCF Division of Pediatric Endocrinology, more than half of all Americans, skinny and fat, have metabolic dysfunction. HALF!

He believes the true epidemic is metabolic syndrome. (6) At the root of an escalating rise in metabolic syndrome is sugar. Particularly fructose. These are a cluster of diseases linked to metabolic syndrome (insulin resistance):

- Diabetes
- Hypertension
- Lipid abnormalities
- Cardiovascular disease
- Non-Alcoholic fatty liver disease
- Polycystic ovarian disease
- Cancer
- Dementia

Wake the Health Up

THE AiR WE BREATHE

Do you know that the air outside your home is likely to be cleaner—less toxic—than the air inside your home?

If we ever hope to have a healthy body, we must stop the daily chemical assault.

When I began my health journey, it started with reading labels on food products. My investigations caused me to wonder how other products were made. Products like my skin care, shampoo, and body lotions. The curiosity expanded to include cleaning products. And then, I heard someone make a comment about the intoxicating "new car smell." It's so inviting—yet so toxic. Again, I said, "What the heck?" Is nothing safe? Nothing and everything are extreme words, but it may be in your health's best interest to buy nothing without doing your due diligence before purchasing anything, and everything. That's a good idea.

Hopefully, paying attention to the chemicals, hormones, and pesticides that flood the food supply helps you understand the benefits of eating clean, toxin-free food. It's time to look at your home environment.

The challenge is that we're surrounded by more than *85,000* environmental toxins and chemicals currently used—or available—in the United States. Many of these chemicals are disruptive to the human body, wildlife, and the environment. Certain chemicals are linked to diseases; brain tumors and leukemia in children, asthma, autism, reproductive problems, and Parkinson's disease are all on the rise. (1)

Again, it's enough to make my head spin. It's clear you must be aware of the toxins you are exposed to, but who has time to check every label? And more importantly, why should you have to spend so much time researching the safety of products? This is where the admonition *"buyer beware"* is good advice. You're the purchaser. You get to decide where to spend your hard-earned money. You choose what you buy. What you eat. What you drink. What skin and body products you apply. What building and decorating supplies you use. What clothes you buy. What furniture you buy. What toys you buy for children. Since you want to make the best possible choices, check the ingredients or materials used in every product you buy for your home and become aware of what impact they have.

Many safe products already exist on the market. They are not the most popular, well-known, or best-advertised brands. Parents, the days are gone when you can give marketers full access to you and to your children. Slick advertising does not guarantee the safety of a product. Know the vision, mission, and the values of any company you regularly give money to in exchange for products.

What products do you use for bath time, and lather on the youngest members of your family? What harsh chemicals are in your cleaning supplies? When I first began to examine the truth behind the fresh, "clean" smell of my laundry detergents and other cleaning supplies, I'll admit I was frustrated. It was almost enough to make me give up trying to clean up my environment. It can be overwhelming. But I knew giving up wasn't the best answer for my health.

Begin your healthy home detox by switching to natural cleaning alternatives. If ingredients are listed, avoid chemicals like ammonia, DEA, APEs, and TEA. If a cleaning product doesn't list ingredients on the label, watch out for words like caution, danger, hazard, or poison on the label.

Natural cleaners may contain small amounts of hard-to-pronounce ingredients. Don't let that deter you! Choose cleaning products with a shorter ingredient list. The best choices include products with plant-based ingredients, followed by solvent-free and phosphate-free labels. Better yet, make your own cleaning products from ingredients typically found in a kitchen: baking soda, lemon, vinegar, and cornstarch are pantry staples that double as effective and safe cleaning products. Hot water and a little elbow grease may be all you need to keep your home environment nice and clean *and healthy.*

Take steps to clean up your body and home from environmental toxins:

1. Avoid PFCs (perfluorochemicals), a class of chemical compounds (PFOA, PFOS, and other per-and polyfluoroalkyl substances). These chemicals are persistent and accumulate in the body and the environment. That means they are not easily metabolized or biodegraded. Studies link these chemicals to adverse health effects including cancer and disruption of thyroid hormone function. (2) PFCs are used to make furniture and carpets stain-resistant, clothing and mattresses water-resistant, furniture and clothing flame retardant, and cookware non-stick. PFCs are also used in some food packaging. (3, 4) Protect your household. Use stainless steel, enameled cast iron, and my favorite...a cast iron skillet. When well-seasoned and carefully cared for, a cast iron skillet is equivalent to non-stick without the added toxins. As you buy clothing, furniture, home goods, and flooring consider how they're made and what materials and chemicals are used in the manufacture.

2. Identify plastic items that contain BPA and phthalates. These man-made chemicals are endocrine disrupters and are connected with a host of health disorders. Although it may be impossible to avoid all plastics, avoid the most dangerous plastics. All plastic containers are marked on the bottom with a number (1-7) in a triangle symbol. Plastics labeled with a 3, 6, or 7 within the triangle are considered the most dangerous. Many manufacturers

proudly list NO BPA in canned foods and plastic ware. That's good news, but I wonder what BPA has been, or will be, replaced with? Refrain from cooking or reheating anything in plastic. Better yet, use glass, stainless steel, or ceramic to store and reheat foods. Phthalates are in personal care items, food packaging, miniblinds, medical equipment, building equipment, and toys. (5, 6, 7)

3. Examine the number of EMFs (electromagnetic fields) emitted by the electrical appliances and wireless devices in your home. It is widely known that air pollution, water contamination, and other environmental toxins can damage health. Data is showing that exposure to EMFs and wireless radiation can synergistically increase the effect of those toxins on the body by damaging the blood-brain barrier. (8) Reduce your exposure by unplugging appliances and devices between uses. Did you just say, "That is too much trouble."? Maybe. Do your research, then decide if you think it is worth the time and effort. Additionally, limit your exposure to EMFs and don't carry your mobile device on your person. (9)

A sampling of how EMF's are emitted:
- Cordless phones
- Wireless baby monitors
- Wireless doorbells
- Wireless routers and modems
- Wireless computers and networks
- Wireless gaming equipment
- Radio

- TV
- Microwave ovens
- X-Rays
- Household appliances
- House wiring
- Powerlines

4. Leave your shoes at the front door. The bottom of footwear is exposed to car oil, pesticides, animal waste, and other toxins. Don't worry about dirt—a little dirt doesn't hurt. But avoid bringing in extra toxins, especially if you have babies crawling or children playing on the floor. Remedy? Place a basket by your front door and fill it with socks or slippers for guests to keep their toes comfy.

5. Get rid of antibacterial and antimicrobial products.

6. Use toxin-free home-building and decorating products.

Chemical companies use you and your children as lab rats without your knowledge or consent. Who will advocate for safe products for you and your children? You must be your own best advocate.

Environmental toxins even have made their way into the womb. More than 230 man-made chemicals have been found in umbilical cords. (10) It's time to stop the onslaught!

There is a ray of hope on the horizon when it comes to the obscene amount of chemicals in use today and the unknown effects on humans, animals, and the environment. The Frank R. Lautenberg Chemical Safety for the 21st Century Act was signed into law June 2016. The Environmental Protection Agency (EPA) is now mandated to evaluate existing chemicals, provide risk-based chemical assessments, and increase public transparency. (11, 12, 13)

History has proven that toxic chemicals, once released into the environment, have the potential to cause long-lasting harm decades after they were "removed." DDT is one example.

I wonder how long the effects of the man-made chemicals in use today will affect the inhabitants of planet earth—birds, animals, me, you, your children, grandchildren, and even great-grandchildren. I pray that chemicals identified as toxic (or potentially toxic) are removed from use promptly—not 30 years down the road. Even so, arm yourself with awareness and do what you can to limit the toxic load.

Here are a few more suggestions to clean up your home environment:
- Grow indoor plants. Lots of them!
- Open your windows and allow fresh air in.
- Open your blinds and let the sunshine in.
- Remove electronics from the bedroom. Or, at a minimum, move them away from the bedside table.
- Recharge your phone a minimum of six feet away from where you recharge your body.

One of the best books I have read on cleaning up the home environment is <u>The Healthy Home</u> by Dr. Myron Wentz and Dave Wentz. This book takes you through each room of your house and gives suggestions for clearing out the potential toxins. I highly recommend it.

Reflect on your current lifestyle behavior:
1. Do you use non-stick cookware? Are there scratch marks in the pan?
2. What types of plastic containers do you use?
3. Do you heat food in plastic?
4. Which, if any, products do you use on your body, or in your home, that have phthalates, BPA's, PFC's, or other harmful chemicals?

Transform your life:
1. What changes will you make to reduce the toxic load inside your home?
2. What will be the biggest challenge for you?
3. How will you overcome that challenge?

TiDY UP!

Does your environment bring you peace and a sense of joy? Or, does it stress you out? Do you keep your home clean, organized, and well maintained, or do you put off cleaning, let the clutter accumulate, and hold on to things long past their usefulness?

Have you heard the saying, "How you do anything, is how you do everything?" The little things may be representative of other patterns. How you take care of your home may be a clue to how you care for your body. As you remove foods that don't serve you, consider clearing out those things taking up extra space in your home—and tidy up the rest. It's incredible how creating space in your home opens up new possibilities in every other area of your life.

If the idea of tidying up your room, home, or office seems overwhelming, work with a professional organizer to get the job done.

If you have already mastered clutter-clearing and you have a workable organizational plan—congratulations! If you struggle with disorganization and hanging on to stuff, I totally get the struggle. I hold on to things way past their usefulness. I grew up in the military and then married into the military. So, I hesitate to let go of some items "because I might need them in my next house." Some items are attached to a special memory. I have all kinds of excuses for hanging on to things, but I discovered the pure joy of cleaning out a drawer or a closet.

If you have items in your home that don't bring you joy, let them go. Gift items to friends or family. Donate unwanted, but useful, items to your favorite charity and let those things bring joy to someone else. If something is broken, ripped, or is flat-out unusable, please don't donate it! Throw the item away!

Managing paper is a biggy for many people. Everyone works differently. I'm a piler. I particularly like to put my piles in baskets. Every basket has a project or a particular focus. It's my system. I know what is in every pile and where each item is in the pile. Just don't move my piles or baskets! If I put something in a file drawer it's out of sight, out of mind. I learned that the hard way. I used to throw mail in a drawer until it was time to make a payment. The due date would come and go, and I would forget. Late fees are stupid tax. It also created a good amount of stress in our lives.

Ray and I had to develop a new system we both can live with. So, we created a designated place for baskets that hold my piles, and we pay bills online. Online banking really cuts down on paper and stress. The baskets are much prettier than piles *and* they are easier to move to a workspace. If you use baskets or plan to, make sure they aren't too deep, or you may spend far too much time digging through the basket to find that ticket, receipt, or file folder.

My system may drive you crazy. Maybe you have a file for everything, and every piece of paper goes in a file folder in a drawer. Or, perhaps you don't do paper at all, and all your filing happens on your computer. Remember, a computer desktop and file folders can be as organized or disorganized as your desk. Create a system that works for you so that you don't create unnecessary *stress* for yourself and spend valuable time searching for a document, a file, or a project.

What are you holding on to? As you clear the joy-sucking items out of your environment, thoroughly clean the area (with natural cleaning products) and enjoy the fruit of your labor. You may be surprised at how much energy you have and find yourself tackling things you have been putting off.

In case you're wondering what clutter has to do with health, imagine how you feel when your desk or home is full of clutter. Clutter can create a drag on mental resources leading to mental fatigue and *stress*. Can you look at a messy pile sitting in the corner and truly enjoy hanging out with friends without feeling guilty or stressed out? Clutter can stagnate the energy in a room and drain your personal energy. Hanging on to old stuff can leave you stuck in the past and unable to make room for the new.

What are you "hanging on to?" How is it impacting your joy and ability to live life to its fullest? Reduce clutter. Reduce stress! Embrace joy!

Reflect on your current lifestyle behavior:
1. What are your current methods of organization in your home? Office?
2. Have you ever missed a tax deduction because the receipt was misplaced?
3. Have you ever paid a late fee because you couldn't find the bill?
4. How do manage paper files? Computer files?
5. Do you buy a stapler, birthday card, or other item only to find the article you already had?
6. Are you a keeper or a sweeper…or somewhere in between?
7. Do you pay for a storage unit?
8. What are you holding on to?
9. Is it easy for you, or a challenge, to sell, toss, or donate items that no longer serve you?

Transform your life:
1. What steps will you take to manage stuff in your life?
2. Which drawer will you clean out first?
3. Where will you donate the stuff you are ready to release?
4. What will you make space for in your life?
5. What will be the biggest challenge for you as you tidy up?
6. How will you overcome that challenge?

HEART OF FORGIVENESS

"You make me so angry!" Have you screamed those words? I have. People get angry. They get hurt by the words or the actions expressed by others. There are countless reasons: a misunderstanding, an unintentional word, an intentional word, an oversight, gossip, an intentionally inflicted hurt, abuse, an affair. Some wounds run very deep.

> **ABOVE ALL ELSE, GUARD YOUR HEART, FOR EVERYTHING YOU DO FLOWS FROM IT.**
> — PROVERBS 4:23 (NiV)

Do you play a scene over and over in your head? You know the one. It's as if you're reliving the moment over and over. Change the channel! When you dwell on anger and replay hurtful, maddening, or painful events over and over, negative emotions fester and grow. Resentment builds. There is nothing righteous about holding onto anger. The toxic effects of holding on to hurt and anger are clinically documented.

At the first sign of anger, stress hormones like cortisol, adrenaline, and noradrenaline kick in to counter the effects of stress. Stress hormones are beneficial for dangerous times but, repeated anger and release of these hormones can create a chain reaction of adverse effects on the body. (1)

Elevated levels of cortisol negatively impact neurons in the prefrontal cortex resulting in poor decision making and future planning. Long periods of elevated stress hormones lead to increased blood glucose, blood pressure, heart rate, pressure on artery walls, and stress-related illness. The hippocampus is also affected by elevated cortisol. The hippocampus—the brain's memory center—is associated with emotions, learning, and memory.

Give yourself time to regroup before you lose your temper. Take deep breaths. Count to ten. Leave the room. Change the conversation. Take control of your anger before it takes control of you.

Serotonin, the happy hormone, is also compromised by too much cortisol. This decrease can result in depression, an increase in aggressive behavior, or heightened feelings of pain and anger. Expressing gratitude increases serotonin production. Actually, an attitude of gratitude has a host of health benefits.

Forgiveness is choosing to let go of resentment. Forgiveness is choosing to express compassion and empathy to the person who wronged you or caused you harm—understanding no one is perfect and that hurt people, hurt people. Sometimes, it's acknowledging your own imperfect behavior. There are times when the person you must forgive is yourself, or you are the one in need of forgiveness.

Benefits of forgiveness:
- Promotes healthier relationships
- Promotes better health and vitality
- Resolves physical symptoms and illness caused by longstanding anger and resentment
- Lowers blood pressure
- Enhances well-being and peace of mind
- Releases bitterness
- Improves sleep patterns
- Increases capacity to love
- Increases ability to trust
- Improves mental health
- Improves self-esteem
- Lessens anxiety and stress
- Reduces anger and hostility

In addition to the physical damage, when you remain angry at someone, you give them power over your thoughts—over you. It doesn't serve you, or your health goals to hang on to anger. Find someone you trust—a confidant, a therapist, a pastor—and begin the healing process. Your mental, physical, and spiritual health depend on it.

Your current pattern of behavior:
1. Do you have unresolved anger you're clinging to?
2. What wrongs have you experienced that you're holding on to?
3. Do you anger easily?
4. What does your angry response look like?
5. Who do you need to forgive?
6. Is it easier for you to forgive or to receive forgiveness?
7. Is there something for which you need forgiveness?
8. How do you typically respond to irritations and frustrations?

Transform your life:
1. What anger, frustration, or hurt will you let go, just for today?
2. What will you do to practice forgiveness?
3. Who do you need to forgive?
4. What will be your biggest challenge?
5. How will you overcome that challenge?

TOO BLESSED TO BE STRESSED!

Stress can be a good thing. Stress response helps protect you from real danger. Unfortunately, that same stress response kicks into action to protect you from *perceived* danger as well.

Although the stress response is meant to protect you from short-term, imminent danger, these days your body's fight or flight mechanism is likely to stay engaged for long periods of time. The brain isn't very intuitive when it comes to distinguishing differences in types of stress to respond appropriately—it senses danger and reacts instantaneously with a fight or flight response. Nerve and hormonal signals jump into action. Your heart rate, blood pressure, and energy level increase to your arms and legs so you can run like the dickens. Cortisol stimulates the release of more glucose (sugar) into the bloodstream for immediate energy AND curbs all unnecessary functions. This means immune, digestive, and reproductive systems are suppressed and won't work while in this state. (1)

Although body systems are designed to return to "normal" duty when the danger has passed, the excessive stress of modern-day life leaves most people in fight or flight mode for long periods of time. This leaves the body to deal with the fallout of chronic stress response. The death of a loved one, a divorce, abuse, and lack of sleep are stressors in the body. Stressful situations in the workplace, at home, in relationships, dealing with finances, and even on the roadways can trigger a stress response. Watching the news—or a scary show—can cause a stress response.

According to the Mayo Clinic, chronic stress exposes the body to an excess of cortisol and other stress hormones and can lead to various health-related problems, including:
- Anxiety
- Depression
- Digestive problems
- Headaches
- Heart disease
- High blood pressure
- Sleep problems
- Build-up of fat tissue
- Weight gain
- Memory and concentration impairment

I look at this list and say, yep, yep, yep! I can see how burning the candle at both ends and multitasking resulted in several of these health issues in my life. It may be impossible to remove all causes of stress from your life, but if you can learn to deal with stressors properly, your body will function better, you'll feel better, and you'll have more clarity.

Implement stress-reducing techniques to reduce the effects of stress on your mind, body, and spirit. Here a few of my favorites:

- Exercise—move the body and stimulate the brain chemicals that promote happiness and relax you. Take a walk and be mindful of your surroundings.
- Implement yoga, or qigong—or tai chi. The movement, deep breathing, and mental focus can bring calm.
- Breathe—deeply from the abdomen!
- Meditation—focus on a calming word.
- Visualize a tranquil place—or your happy place.
- Eat well—of course, a healthy diet is beneficial! Eat a healthy anti-inflammatory diet full of high-quality proteins, leafy greens and vegetables, and healthy fats.
- Sleep—review "Get Your Z's" if you need a refresher.
- Gratitude—identify people, places, events, and things for which you are grateful and express some form of gratitude daily.
- Laughter—laughter is the best medicine! Some of my favorite memories are those shared with friends when spontaneous laughter erupted throughout the room. I especially love the snorting laughter because—let's be honest—who can resist laughing at a snort. A good belly laugh requires deep breaths which stimulates your heart, lungs, and muscles. It's almost like a workout! Your brain also releases endorphins—that feel-good hormone—while you're laughing.
- Plan your Life! Organize your work and living spaces. Plan your schedule. Use any type of calendar that you will actually use. I use a physical planner for big-picture

planning and the calendar in my phone to track daily commitments. Find a system that works for you and implement it. Prioritize tasks and concentrate on one task at a time. I used to think I was good at multitasking. I know now I was deceiving myself. Here's the big challenge: delegate tasks that you aren't equipped for or skilled at, or you don't have the time to do. Don't forget to plan in playtime, exercise, and other activities central to your personal growth and development.

Reflect on your current lifestyle behavior:
1. Where does stress show up in your life?
2. How do you respond to stress?
3. What keeps you up at night?
4. What do you worry about?
5. Which stressors are imagined? Which are real?
6. Are you an optimist, or a pessimist?
7. Do you have a confidant?
8. On a scale of 1-10 how content are you with your life?

Transform your life:
1. Identify stressors which you have control over. What will you do to alter the source of stress?
2. What will you do to alter your reaction to stressors you can't control?
3. What activities can you use to relieve stress?
4. What will be your biggest challenge?
5. How will you overcome that challenge?

GiVE YOURSELF SOME LOVE

Maybe by now, you've noticed a recurring theme. Developing habits that include quality sleep, managing stress, eating nourishing food, drinking adequate water, moving the body, and tending to your needs beyond the plate is a solution to most of the topics addressed in this book. These habits are the ultimate in self-care, self-love. In fact, I hope you see that they all work synergistically and are vital to optimal health care.

Self-care isn't a luxury. Self-care isn't self-indulgent or self-centered. It's a necessity. Self-care is vital to wellbeing. How can you possibly give your best when you're not at your best? If you're not adequately nourished (emotionally, physically, or spiritually), it's impossible to give to others from a place of love, contribution, abundance—overflow.

Yet, there are acts of self-care that can be neglected, and over time the neglect impacts overall health. Self-care is maintaining a healthy relationship with yourself. It's about deliberately choosing activities to care for your mental, emotional, and physical health. Self-care is something that fills you up—not something that drains you. Self-care might just be a simple act of just *being*. Life is hectic—who has time to rest, to play, to just *be*? Take time!

When you are spiritually, emotionally, or physically depleted, your interactions with family, friends, or clients may come from a place of resentment and stress. Self-care is about bringing a sense of peace and wellbeing to your mind and body. Another way to think of self-care is taking time to decompress, to renew, to restore your sense of self.

Self-care is an activity that nurtures and refuels you on a deep level. Maybe it's a soothing bath, or a refreshing shower, a mani-pedi, getting a haircut, or a shave. What nurtures and refuels you will be as individualized as your dietary and exercise needs.

What does self-care look like?
1. Choose food that nourishes you.
2. Stay hydrated. Water is essential.
3. Commit to seven to nine hours of quality sleep every night.
4. Breathe. Breathe again.
5. Forgive, quickly.
6. Move your body. Find an activity that invigorates you and that you genuinely enjoy. Dance like no one is watching—shake your booty! Take a yoga or Pilates class. Swim, bowl, play tennis. Avoid sitting for long periods of time.
7. Get outside and connect with nature. Get 15 minutes of sunlight every day.

8. Sit on a park bench. Find a swing. Lounge on your front porch or in your backyard…let your mind wander. Just BE.
9. Take a walk—or a run. Take your dog along if you have one.
10. Take a hike in the mountains.
11. Play in the dirt. Plant a garden, a flower, or a tree—connect with nature. Get grounded!
12. Hit the beach, walk in the sand, take in the smell of the ocean water and the feel of the ocean breeze.
13. Write in your journal 5-15 minutes a day. Pen to paper.
14. Create more joy. Develop an attitude of gratitude. Every day write down:
    - Three things you're grateful for
    - Three people you're grateful for
15. Dedicate time daily for spiritual practice. Meditate or pray.
16. Implement a new spiritual practice.
17. Do something nice for someone else—just because.
18. Schedule a massage or trade back rubs with a close friend.
19. Take a bath—light a candle. Add in essential oils and Epsom salts.*
20. Play!
21. Listen to music—soft and low or loud and raucous.
22. Turn off technology for one hour…or a whole day.
23. Take a nap.
24. Paint, sketch, or capture moments through photography.
25. Read a novel or a magazine.
26. Plan a day out with a pal. Lunch, movie, coffee, laugh, be!

27. Call a friend.
28. Snuggle with your honey.
29. Laugh every day. On purpose. Laugh some more.
30. Color (Yes, color! There are tons of adult coloring books—get one!)
31. Declutter a drawer.
32. Tackle something on your bucket list.

Add your own self-care ideas to this list:

33._____

34._____

35._____

Which practices from the above list (especially the ones you added to the list) make you say, "I wish" ... "if only" ... "I don't have time for that" ... "That will be the day." Write those down! Add one or two of these self-care practices to your schedule. Be intentional. Pick those that will nourish your spirit and bring you a sense of joy.

Reflect on your current lifestyle behavior:
1. In what ways do you currently practice self-care?
2. Which self-care practices fill you up?
3. What makes you feel grounded and well cared for?
4. In what ways do you neglect yourself?
5. In what way is your body screaming for attention?

Transform your life:
1. What would your life look like if you took more time for self-care?
2. Which self-care practice(s) will you integrate into your regular routine?
3. What will be the biggest challenge for you?
4. How will you overcome that challenge?

*** Reap detoxing health benefits with Epson Salts**
A soak in the bathtub can be more than an activity (however blissful) to unwind, relax, and detoxify emotions. Throw in some Epsom salts and reap the nourishing and detoxifying health benefits of an Epsom salt bath: relax your muscles, reduce inflammation, loosen stiff joints and pull toxins from your body. Magnesium and sulfate (mineral compounds in Epsom salts) are absorbed by the skin and used by the body's detoxification pathways, to neutralize toxins, and to excrete heavy metals. As a bonus, an Epsom salt bath will stimulate movement in the colon as part of the detox process. You may feel more relaxed and sleep better.

Add one to two cups of Epsom salts to *warm* water, swish to dissolve the salt, slide in, soak for 12 to 15 minutes and reap the health benefits. Step out without using soap or rinsing off and towel dry. Add 5-10 drops of essential oil for additional benefit. Grapefruit, rosemary, lemon, lavender, and frankincense are my favorites. Optional: add equal amounts of baking soda and Epsom salts.

SUPPLEMENTS... ARE NOT REPLACEMENTS!

When I was clearing out *old* paperwork, I found a note from the mid-1990's that my doctor at the time wrote on a prescription pad. It listed the name of a pharmaceutical vitamin company and her recommendation of what products I should take. At the time, I was facing multiple health challenges, my energy was non-existent, and I lived in a state of depression. Blood tests showed my levels of B-vitamins were extremely low. She gave me a B-12 shot to give my body an immediate boost. Wow! What a difference that dose of vitamin B-12 made in my life! During this time, my body was desperately trying to get my attention. Knock, knock, knock. I wasn't paying attention. Looking back, now, I can clearly see the warning signs that led up to that emergency gallbladder surgery. I was carrying around an extra 75 pounds, yet I was nutrient deficient and virtually every system in my body was screaming for help. As it turned out, the pharmaceutical vitamin company my doctor jotted down on that prescription pad was the same company my friend introduced me to more than a decade later. I wonder what could have been different in my health journey if I had followed my doctor's wise recommendation those many years earlier. Although I can't go back in time, I'm eternally grateful that my friend cared enough about me, and the health struggles I was going through, to introduce me to a solution. I have reclaimed my health and vitality, as a result.

The human body is designed to be fueled and nourished by the vitamins, minerals, fats, proteins, and carbohydrates in our food. In a perfect world (and perfect digestion) we'd get all the nutrients we need from our food. Not many of us are perfect.

I know I need 9-13 servings of fruits and vegetables every day. I know I need to get 7½ to 8 hours of sleep every night. I know I need to move my body every day. I know I need fresh air and sunshine every day. I know, I know, I know. Yet, I don't live in a perfect world. And you probably don't either. I do the best I can as often as I can. Even though I know what to eat, there are times when I go several days in a row without the recommended servings of fruits and vegetables. There are days when I eat at a restaurant that may not serve the highest quality food. There are days when I drink too much coffee. There are days my stress level is out of control. There are days when I don't get enough sleep. Additionally, I'm still healing from the consequences of a leaky gut, and my body is bombarded every day with environmental toxins. So, I choose to take vitamin and mineral supplements to help my body get adequate nutrition.

If you suspect you have digestive issues, begin healing your gut and work with a professional to determine which supplements will best support your healing process. If your digestion is compromised, you won't receive the full benefit of a nutritional supplement, even if it's the highest quality supplement on the market.

"Supplement" is the operative word. Supplements aren't a substitute for eating healthy foods and developing better lifestyle habits. They're meant to fill in the gap. Again, most people these days have quite a few gaps.

Like every other topic we have discussed, scientists and experts have differing opinions about whether nutritional supplements are warranted, or not. The discussion includes which form, or brand, is best. There are many good-quality supplements on the market. Do your research. Supplements are not all created equal.

Wake the Health Up

FiNAL THOUGHTS

Have you woke the health up?

The information I've shared with you in this book is the tip of the iceberg. There is so much more to say, to learn, about how the body functions and what steps we can take to create a body that thrives. I pray you are inspired to continue your journey to health.

Hopefully, by now, you are well on your way to a lifestyle overhaul, a fresh mind, and a revitalized body.

Here's a review:

- Remove—Toxic chemicals, inflammatory foods and beverages, toxic relationships, toxic thoughts, and habits that don't serve you. Skip antibacterial anything.

- Replace—Eat clean, organic, healthy (for you) nutrient-rich food. Get picky about your personal care products too. Spend time with people, places, and things that bring you joy. Express gratitude. Drink lots of water.

- Reinoculate—Consume a healthy balance of good bacteria with a quality multi-strain probiotic. Eat prebiotic foods that feed the good bacteria. Eat lots of leafy greens. Use a high-quality supplement to fill the gaps in your diet.

- Ruminate—Chew your food. While you're at it, don't forget to breathe before you eat. Be mindful of what you are eating. Be mindful of the blessings and the challenges in your life (because they are blessings as well). And give that "eating window" thing a try.

- Repair—Improve your gut health; increase fresh whole fruits, vegetables, chia seeds, bone broth, prebiotic foods (kefir, sauerkraut, fermented foods), digestive enzymes and liver support supplements. Oh, and get your sleep.

- Rev up your life—Move 30 minutes a day, doing whatever movement makes you happy. Stop sitting around! Get that lymphatic system going. Develop a few muscles—they don't have to be bulging!

- Restore—Set aside a minimum of 30 minutes every day to do something for you and no one else—something that fills you with joy. Connect with yourself. Put your thoughts in writing every day. Connect with the outdoors: walk in the grass, play in the dirt. Heal and let go of past emotional wounds. Engage in spiritual practices. Set aside time to do something for others.

- Read—Be an informed consumer. Become an avid label reader. Hopefully by now you know why.

If your health isn't where you want it to be—yet—that's okay. Take baby steps. Keep making changes. Add in those things that will create a healthier you. Read this book again. Review your responses to the questions in this book and celebrate the progress you are make. I hope I have inspired you to seek answers to your health-related questions. Stay curious!

Your health will transform as you adopt new healthy habits. One day you will wake up and realize these habits are a "normal" part of your new lifestyle.

You don't have to do this alone. Lean on supportive family and friends. Seek a certified health coach to help guide you on your journey. Find a coach that's a good match for you and your specific health goals.

It's your body. Love it or leave it. No one gets out of this life alive; every one of us will die—sooner or later. I prefer it to be later. Living here on earth or going home to glory are both a win. How you live—your quality of life—makes all the difference. The body is a magnificent and intricately designed machine, and it will support you in living out your dreams and your purpose when it is properly cared for.

May you live life in happiness and health all the days of your life!

ACKNOWLEDGEMENTS

My heart overflows with gratitude for the incredible people who love me, encourage me, inspire me, prompt me, challenge me, and cheer me on. This book began with a glimmer of a thought, and without them, this book would still be just a dream. Words cannot adequately express the immense gratitude I have for each person involved in every stage of writing, editing, and publishing of this work. In addition to those listed below, I am also grateful for Missy and Fred Day, Angela Gardner, Alan Ashford, Alicia Mejia, Cheryl Barnes and my community of friends. I want to list every single one of you!

Thank you, Neal and Dorothy Portnoy, for the conversation around the kitchen table that formed the title of this book.

Erin Nausin, I am in awe of your creative spirit. Your design for the cover captures the essence of "Wake the Health Up!" I am sincerely grateful for your partnership in this project.

Janice Demaree, Lynne Cavalieri, Jen Anderson, Nancy Ashford, Nancy Gabriel, Faye Bastarache, and Mia Watler, I am beyond grateful for your unwavering support and the hours you spent around the kitchen table, in the coffee shop, and at your own computers, throughout the many stages of the writing and editing process. Your support, encouragement, contribution, collaboration, and editing skills left fingerprints on this work. Your sacrifice and your contribution to this project almost leave me speechless.

Karen Langston, thank you for igniting my desire to learn the connection between digestion and health. I am deeply grateful for your contribution as the content editor and for writing the foreword. You continue to inspire me to dive deep into the study of gut health. Oh, and thank you for making poop my favorite four-letter word!

Michelle (Poe) Hausbeck, you took a concept in my head, Erin's cover design, and your own brand of ingenuity and brought life to the contents of this book as the Layout and Content Designer.

I am grateful for Joshua Rosenthal and the Institute for Integrative Nutrition (IIN) for broadening my view of what it means to be healthy and that the road to health is unique for each person. I am grateful for my IIN classmates who have been on this journey with me, especially Julie Amsden, Lauren Bahr, and Joan Kero. You inspire me.

And I am grateful for the gift of my family: for my parents, Mickey and Del Hagen who planted love, faith, and a sense of contribution in me at a young age; for my daughter, Lyndsay Betts, son-in-law, Ryan Rouse, and my grandson Kenny and his family, Tricia, and Asher Barron who inspire me to be my healthiest self.

I am eternally grateful for my husband, Ray, and his undying, unconditional love, and encouragement. Ray, your insight throughout the writing process was invaluable. And I am so grateful that you kept us fed and in clean clothes. I love doing life with you!

Wake the Health Up

RECiPES

As a young cook, I followed a recipe exactly. I wouldn't deviate even ¼ of a teaspoon. I became a cookbook and online recipe addict. As my love of cooking developed, I gained the confidence to become more creative in combining foods and spices to my taste.

I still love cookbooks. Sometimes it's necessary to follow recipes exactly (especially with baking). But I typically use recipes as inspiration. I read the recipes, get an idea of the ingredients, and then I adapt. I peruse cookbooks for hours—then go make my own creation.

Then there are times I get in the kitchen and get creative with the ingredients I have on hand. I throw in a little of this and a little of that.

I love to use new spices and to experiment with flavor combinations. That's how I come up with some of our favorite dishes. Here are a few recipes to get your creativity flowing. Play—experiment—with your food. Discover new spices.

BUTTERNUT SQUASH AND CARROT CURRY SOUP

One day I had butternut squash and carrots on hand. It was Fall, and I was hungry for soup. I roasted the cubed butternut squash and carrots and added a few more ingredients and created a yummy soup. This is what I added:

Cut one butternut squash and 3 large carrots into 1" chunks. Toss with coconut oil, sea salt, and pepper.

Roast at 400 degrees until very tender—30-40 minutes.

In a Dutch oven, sauté a red onion for a few minutes and then add in a diced peeled green apple and cook just until tender.

Add spices. This is what I used: 2-3 teaspoons of grated ginger, about a 1/2 teaspoon of freshly grated nutmeg, 2 teaspoons of cinnamon, 2 teaspoons curry powder, salt and pepper. Experiment with which spices and how much of each you prefer.

Add the roasted squash and carrots. Stir in three to four cups organic vegetable (or chicken) broth and heat through.

Use an immersion blender and blend the soup until smooth.

Stir in 14 ounces of coconut milk. Heat through on a gentle simmer.

Sprinkle the top with pumpkin seeds. And dig in!

This soup was yummy the first night, but the second day was awesome!

Enjoy!!

BEET, GOAT CHEESE AND KALE SALAD

- 1 bunch of kale, washed and dried and torn (or chopped) in bite-sized pieces
- Goat cheese (optional)
- 1/2 to 2/3 cup roughly chopped whole almonds
- 1/3 to 1/2 cup Goji berries or cranberries
- 3-4 roasted and diced beets depending on the size of the beets (Costco sells cooked organic beets if you want a quicker option)
- 1/3 to 1/2 cup of a vinaigrette-based dressing (recipes to follow).

Place kale in a large bowl.

Pour half the dressing on the kale and using your impeccably clean hands make sure all the kale pieces are covered. Add more dressing, if necessary.

Add the berries and beets. Add a bit more dressing if you want. Toss the ingredients together. Place in the refrigerator.

When ready to serve, add the almonds and goat cheese. Slightly toss to mix ingredients.

Serve and enjoy!

CRANBERRY, BLUE CHEESE AND KALE SALAD

- 1 bunch of kale, washed and dried and torn (or chopped) in bite-sized pieces
- Toasted coarsely chopped walnuts (Heat dry skillet and "toast" the nuts—watch them carefully). Or substitute your favorite nut or seed.
- ½ cup dried cranberries (without added sugar, or sweetened with fruit juice)
- 1 large or 2 small green apples diced in 1/4" chunks
- 1/2 a red onion, cut in thin slivers
- Crumpled blue cheese
- 1/3 to 1/2 cup of a vinaigrette-based dressing (recipes to follow).

Place kale in a large bowl.

Pour half the dressing on the kale and using your impeccably clean hands make sure all the kale pieces are covered. Add more dressing, if necessary.

Add cranberries, diced apples, sliced onions, and blue cheese. Add a bit more dressing if you want. Place in the refrigerator.

When ready to serve add, the blue cheese and toasted walnuts.

Salads can be a healthy meal or side dish. A quick look at a restaurant menu that includes calories can be eye-opening. Often, the calorie count for a "healthy-looking" salad exceeds the 1,000 calorie mark. Dressings may be one of the reasons.

It is difficult to know the ingredients in a restaurant dressing. Store-bought dressings do have a label, and that label often reveals inflammatory oils, sugar, artificial flavors, preservatives, and MSG. Read the labels on dressings in your pantry or refrigerator. What do you see? Do you understand each ingredient and its purpose?

DRESSiNGS

Making your own dressing isn't just tasty, it's the best way to ensure quality ingredients. Making your own dressing is also cheaper than buying store-bought dressings. Once you get the basics down, experiment with a variety of bases, oils, acids, and spices to create dressings.

A BASIC VINAIGRETTE

Use a ratio of 3 to 1, or equal parts of a healthy oil and an acid—or somewhere in the middle—depending on the acid and the flavor you want. Use a good quality extra virgin olive oil and a healthy acid such as fresh lemon, lime, or orange, raw organic apple cider vinegar, aged balsamic vinegar. Add sea salt, pepper, herbs, and spices to taste. That's it!

VINAIGRETTE FOR KALE SALAD

In a jar mix together:
- 1/3 cup apple cider vinegar
- 1/2 cup olive oil
- 2 to 6 tablespoons of dijon mustard— depending on the taste and consistency you want
- 1 teaspoon of maple syrup or honey, optional
- Sea salt and freshly ground pepper, to taste

Shake well—about 20 to 25 seconds. I usually make this dressing as I need it, but you can make it ahead and store it 3 to 4 days.

CREAMY RANCH-STYLE DRESSING

- 1/4 cup high-quality mayonnaise (or make your own)
- 3/4 cup organic Greek yogurt
- 1/4 cup coconut milk
- 1 1/2 teaspoons Bragg's apple cider vinegar
- 3/4 teaspoon onion powder
- 3/4 teaspoon garlic powder
- 1 tablespoon finely chopped fresh dill or 1 teaspoon dried dill.
- Salt and pepper, to taste.

Whisk together the mayo, yogurt, coconut milk, and apple cider vinegar. Stir in the spices. Adjust seasonings and add more coconut milk for the taste and consistency you want. This is best made a day ahead to allow the flavors to marry.

Alternative: Use almond milk or organic half n half in place of the coconut milk.

HONEY MUSTARD, KALE, AND ROSEMARY CHICKEN

- 1/2 cup grainy mustard, or dijon—or go wild and use half of each.
- 1/4 cup honey or maple syrup
- 1 small onion, diced
- 2 or 3 garlic cloves, minced
- 2 fresh rosemary sprigs—strip rosemary from the stem
- 6-8 boneless, skinless chicken thighs
- Ghee
- 1 bunch of kale, strip from the stem, roll the leaves together and cut into thin strips (or chop the kale, or keep the kale leaves whole—it's entirely up to you). Swiss chard works well in this recipe as well.

Step 1: Combine the mustard and the honey (or maple syrup) and set it aside.

Step 2: In an oven-proof pan, sauté the onion in ghee for a couple of minutes and then add 2 or 3 minced garlic cloves. Don't add the garlic too soon, or it will brown and get bitter. Push the onion mixture aside and brown the chicken on both sides…add a bit more ghee, if necessary.

If you want to add greens to your diet (I know you do!) go to step 3. If you haven't wholly embraced cooked greens yet, skip step 3.

Step 3: Remove the chicken from the pan and stir in chopped kale or, swiss chard. Cook the greens a few minutes. Salt and pepper to taste. Place the chicken on top of the cooked greens in the same pan.

Step 4: Pour the honey and mustard mixture over the chicken and sprinkle with the rosemary.

Step 5: Bake covered at 400 degrees for 15 minutes. Remove the lid and baste the chicken with the honey mustard sauce in the pan and cook uncovered with an additional 10 to 20 minutes (depending on the type of chicken you used) or until done.

Add a salad or a side of quinoa and enjoy.

CHiCKEN CHiLi

- 1 tablespoon avocado oil
- 1 1/2 pounds cooked, cubed boneless, skinless chicken breasts or thighs
- 1/2 cup chopped onion
- 2 cloves garlic, finely minced
- 1 small red bell pepper, diced
- 1 jalapeño, diced (use seeds and veins if you want spicy)
- 32 ounces organic chicken broth
- 1/2 teaspoon salt
- 1/2 teaspoon pepper
- 1/2 teaspoon dried oregano
- 1 to 2 teaspoons chili powder
- 1/2 to 1 teaspoon coriander
- 1 tablespoon cumin
- 1/2 to 1 teaspoon paprika
- 2 cans (15-ounces each) white beans (like Great Northern or cannoli beans), rinsed and drained
- Organic BPA-free canned (or jarred) roasted tomatoes
- Juice of 1 lime
- 1/2 cup chopped fresh cilantro

Heat the oil in a large pot, and add the onion, red bell pepper, jalapeño pepper, and garlic. Sauté for 3-4 minutes or until the veggies begin to soften.

Stir in the cumin, salt, pepper, oregano, and chili powder, coriander, paprika and lightly toast the spices in the bottom of the pot. I don't measure. I use the palm of my hand or the lid of the spice jar. Start with a smaller measurement of each spice and adjust the amount to your taste.

Stir in the chicken broth. Make sure you scrape all the yummy goodness off the bottom of the pan. Add the chicken, beans, and tomatoes.

Simmer for about 30 minutes until beans and broth are heated through.

Stir in the lime and cilantro. Adjust the salt and pepper to taste.

Serve it up with diced avocado and more chopped cilantro for extra yumminess.

HOMEMADE CHiCKEN BONE BROTH

- Boned chicken carcass (skin, bones, neck, etc.)
- 1 onion, quartered
- 2 large carrots, cut in half
- 2 stalks celery, cut in half (with some leaves)
- 3-5 garlic cloves, slightly mashed
- 1 teaspoon thyme or 3-4 fresh sprigs
- 1 teaspoon parsley or 4-5 sprigs
- 1 teaspoon oregano
- 1 teaspoon Himalayan sea salt
- 1 teaspoons peppercorns
- 2-3 tablespoons apple cider vinegar

Combine the ingredients in the pot; Cover with filtered water and bring to a boil. You can use a crock pot or cook the broth low and slow on the stovetop.

Reduce to a simmer for 8 to 36 hours. Add more water as necessary. The longer the broth cooks, the more the minerals are pulled from the bones.

Strain and discard everything from the broth. Enjoy!

*Use organic vegetables and organic humanly-raised poultry to receive the best health benefits of bone broth.

Bone broth is excellent for sipping, especially when sick or you have tummy issues. The bone broth can also be used in other recipes. Store in the refrigerator up to three days. Freeze recipe-sized portions, in glass or BPA and phthalate-free plastic, once broth has cooled.

REFERENCES

The Root of It!
1. https://www.aarda.org/diseaselist/
2. https://www.cdc.gov/chronicdisease/about/index.htm
3. https://my.clevelandclinic.org/health/transcripts/1444_lifestyle-choices-root-causes-of-chronic-diseases
4. https://www.cdc.gov/chronicdisease/about/costs/index.htm
5. https://www.cdc.gov/healthyschools/chronicconditions.htm
6. https://www.ncbi.nlm.nih.gov/pmc/articles/PMC3492709/
7. Quote by Benjamin Franklin: "An ounce of prevention is …. https://www.goodreads.com/quotes/247269-an-ounce-of-prevention-is-worth-a-pound-of-cure

On the Inside Tract
1. https://www.ncbi.nlm.nih.gov/pmc/articles/PMC3983973/
2. https://www.niddk.nih.gov/health-information/health-statistics/digestive-diseases
3. https://www.ncbi.nlm.nih.gov/pmc/articles/PMC3492709/
4. https://www.ncbi.nlm.nih.gov/pmc/articles/PMC5772764/
5. https://nutritionreview.org/2018/03/gastric-balance-heartburn-caused-excess-acid/
6. https://www.ncbi.nlm.nih.gov/pmc/articles/PMC5440529/

7. https://www.ncbi.nlm.nih.gov/pubmed/22109896
8. https://hypothyroidmom.com/zonulin-leaky-gut-gluten-autoimmune-disease-thyroid-this-pioneering-researcher-tells-all/

Clean It Up, Clear It Out.
1. https://www.ncbi.nlm.nih.gov/pmc/articles/PMC3879711/
2. https://www.ncbi.nlm.nih.gov/pmc/articles/PMC3106288/ and https://www.ncbi.nlm.nih.gov/pmc/articles/PMC3389582/
3. http://www.vivo.colostate.edu/hbooks/pathphys/digestion/stomach/mmcomplex.html

Honey, We Have Company!
1. https://www.ncbi.nlm.nih.gov/pmc/articles/PMC3709439/
2. https://www.ncbi.nlm.nih.gov/pmc/articles/PMC4191858/
3. https://www.hmpdacc.org/overview/
4. https://en.wikipedia.org/wiki/Human_Microbiome_Project
5. https://www.nih.gov/news-events/news-releases/nih-human-microbiome-project-defines-normal-bacterial-makeup-body
6. https://www.ncbi.nlm.nih.gov/pmc/articles/PMC2643114/
7. https://www.ncbi.nlm.nih.gov/pmc/articles/PMC4303825/
8. https://www.ncbi.nlm.nih.gov/pmc/articles/PMC6033410/
9. https://journals.plos.org/plosone/article?id=10.1371/journal.pone.0199899
10. https://www.ncbi.nlm.nih.gov/pmc/articles/PMC2643114/
11. https://www.ncbi.nlm.nih.gov/pmc/articles/PMC2631814/
12. https://www.fda.gov/NewsEvents/Newsroom/PressAnnouncements/ucm517478.htm

About Antibiotics...
1. https://www.cdc.gov/features/antibioticuse/index.html
2. https://www.cdc.gov/antibiotic-use/
3. https://www.ncbi.nlm.nih.gov/pubmed/16696665
4. https://www.ncbi.nlm.nih.gov/pmc/articles/PMC4259177/

Move It, Move It, Move It!
1. http://annals.org/aim/article-abstract/2091327/sedentary-time-its-association-risk-disease-incidence-mortality-hospitalization-adults

Get Your Z's The Body is Up to Something Good!
1. https://www.ncbi.nlm.nih.gov/books/NBK19961/ and https://www.cdc.gov/sleep/data_statistics.html
2. https://newsinhealth.nih.gov/2013/04/sleep-it
3. https://www.ncbi.nlm.nih.gov/pmc/articles/PMC3389582/
4. https://www.google.com/amp/s/www.thesleepdoctor.com/2017/11/15/truth-alcohol-sleep/amp/
5. https://www.scientificamerican.com/article/q-a-why-is-blue-light-before-bedtime-bad-for-sleep/

Eat Clean?
1. https://www.nongmoproject.org/gmo-facts/
2. https://www.nongmoproject.org/gmo-facts/
3. http://www.iarc.fr/en/media-centre/iarcnews/pdf/MonographVolume112.pdf
4. https://www.p65warnings.ca.gov/sites/default/files/downloads/factsheets/glyphosate_fact_sheet.pdf
5. https://www.ecowatch.com/roundup-cancer-1882187755.html

6. https://www.usda.gov/media/blog/2013/05/17/organic-101-can-gmos-be-used-organic-products
7. https://www.ams.usda.gov/sites/default/files/media/OrganicLabelsExplained.png
8. https://www.ams.usda.gov/sites/default/files/media/BehindTheUSDAOrganicSeal.png
9. http://www.ams.usda.gov/sites/default/files/media/BehindTheUSDAOrganicSeal.png

Let's Get Cooking!
1. https://www.fda.gov/food/labelingnutrition/ucm436722.htm
2. https://pubs.acs.org/doi/abs/10.1021/acs.jafc.7b03118?source=cen
3. https://foodrevolution.org/blog/how-to-wash-vegetables-fruits/#wash
4. https://www.ncbi.nlm.nih.gov/pubmed/16635908   and https://www.ncbi.nlm.nih.gov/pmc/articles/PMC3384703/
5. https://www.ncbi.nlm.nih.gov/pubmed/24689456
6. https://www.ncbi.nlm.nih.gov/pubmed/29662290
7. https://www.ncbi.nlm.nih.gov/pubmed/20868314

Go Green! Red, Purple, Orange and Yellow Too!
1. https://www.ncbi.nlm.nih.gov/pmc/articles/PMC5452159/
2. https://www.ncbi.nlm.nih.gov/pubmed/22364157
3. https://www.ncbi.nlm.nih.gov/pmc/articles/PMC5452159/
4. https://academic.oup.com/ajcn/article/95/2/454/4576804
5. http://www.aicr.org/cancer-research-update/2012/december_5_2012/cru-flavonoids-prevention.html

A Grain of Salt with a Side of Iodine

1. McMaster University. "Pass the salt: Study finds average consumption safe for heart health: Public health strategies should be based on best evidence." ScienceDaily. ScienceDaily, 9 August 2018. https://www.sciencedaily.com/releases/2018/08/180809202057.htm
2. https://www.ncbi.nlm.nih.gov/pubmed/21036373
3. https://www.ncbi.nlm.nih.gov/pubmed/21731062
4. https://www.ncbi.nlm.nih.gov/pmc/articles/PMC5179550/
5. https://www.heart.org/en/news/2018/07/17/experts-criticize-new-study-about-salt-consumption
6. https://www.ncbi.nlm.nih.gov/pmc/articles/PMC3074887/
7. https://www.mdedge.com/ccjm/article/132156/endocrinology/iodine-deficiency-clinical-implications
8. https://ods.od.nih.gov/factsheets/Iodine-HealthProfessional/

Gimme Coffee!

1. https://health.usnews.com/wellness/for-parents/articles/2017-06-01/caffeine-a-growing-problem-for-children
2. https://www.researchgate.net/publication/279923885_Effects_of_caffeine_on_health_and_nutrition_A_Review and https://www.ncbi.nlm.nih.gov/pubmed/18606630
3. https://www.researchgate.net/publication/279923885_Effects_of_caffeine_on_health_and_nutrition_A_Review
4. https://www.precisionnutrition.com/coffee-and-hormones
5. https://www.researchgate.net/publication/279923885_Effects_of_caffeine_on_health_and_nutrition_A_Review

6. https://www.precisionnutrition.com/coffee-and-hormones
7. https://www.webmd.com/vitamins/ai/ingredientmono-979/caffeine
8. https://www.researchgate.net/publication/279923885_Effects_of_caffeine_on_health_and_nutrition_A_Review and https://www.precisionnutrition.com/coffee-and-hormones.
9. https://www.researchgate.net/publication/279923885_Effects_of_caffeine_on_health_and_nutrition_A_Review
10. https://www.eurekalert.org/pub_releases/2016-06/aaos-chl061316.php

What's in a Label?

1. https://www.ncbi.nlm.nih.gov/pmc/articles/PMC6033410/
2. https://s3.amazonaws.com/public-inspection.federalregister.gov/2015-14883.pdf
3. https://www.fda.gov/Food/IngredientsPackagingLabeling/FoodAdditivesIngredients/ucm449162.htm
4. https://www.fda.gov/Food/ucm292278.htm
5. https://www.accessdata.fda.gov/scripts/cdrh/cfdocs/cfcfr/CFRSearch.cfm?FR=180.30
6. https://www.scientificamerican.com/article/soda-chemical-cloudy-health-history/
7. https://www.scientificamerican.com/article/bha-and-bht-a-case-for-fresh/
8. https://www.ncbi.nlm.nih.gov/books/NBK209859/
9. https://www.fda.gov/Food/GuidanceRegulation/GuidanceDocumentsRegulatoryInformation/LabelingNutrition/ucm385663.htm
10. https://www.ncbi.nlm.nih.gov/pubmed/18783640

Speaking of Sugar
1. https://health.clevelandclinic.org/polycystic-ovary-syndrome-pill-not-remedy/
2. http://sugarscience.ucsf.edu/the-growing-concern-of-overconsumption.html
3. https://www.ncbi.nlm.nih.gov/pubmed/16460879/
4. https://www.medicalnewstoday.com/articles/282604.php?sr
5. https://www.ncbi.nlm.nih.gov/pmc/articles/PMC2660468/
6. https://www.ncbi.nlm.nih.gov/pmc/articles/PMC3772345/
7. https://www.fda.gov/Food/IngredientsPackagingLabeling/FoodAdditivesIngredients/ucm397716.htm

Obesity…It's an Epidemic!
1. https://stateofobesity.org/healthcare-costs-obesity/
2. https://www.marketresearch.com/Marketdata-Enterprises-Inc-v416/Weight-Loss-Diet-Control-10825677/
3. https://stateofobesity.org/rates/
4. https://www.cdc.gov/obesity/data/adult.html
5. https://stateofobesity.org/data/
6. http://youtu.be/ceFyF9px20Y

The Air We Breathe
1. https://www.edf.org/sites/default/files/specialreport_spring2015.pdf
2. https://www.epa.gov/pfas/basic-information-pfas#health
3. https://www.niehs.nih.gov/health/materials/perflourinated_chemicals_508.pdf
4. https://www.epa.gov/pfas/basic-information-pfas#health
5. https://www.pehsu.net/_Library/facts/bpapatients_factsheet03-2014.pdf

6. https://toxtown.nlm.nih.gov/chemicals-and-contaminants/phthalates
7. https://www.cdc.gov/biomonitoring/Phthalates_FactSheet.html
8. https://ehtrust.org/key-issues/the-environment-and-health/wireless-radiationelectromagnetic-fields-increases-toxic-body-burden/
9. https://www.powerwatch.org.uk/elf/overview.asp
10. https://www.edf.org/sites/default/files/specialreport_spring2015.pdf
11. https://www.epa.gov/assessing-and-managing-chemicals-under-tsca/frank-r-lautenberg-chemical-safety-21st-century-act
12. https://www.epa.gov/newsreleases/epa-marks-chemical-safety-milestone-1st-anniversary-lautenberg-chemical-safety-act
13. https://www.epa.gov/assessing-and-managing-chemicals-under-tsca/frank-r-lautenberg-chemical-safety-21st-century-act-5

Heart of Forgiveness
1. https://www.iahe.com/docs/articles/nicabm-anger-infographic-printable-pdf.pdf
2. https://www.hopkinsmedicine.org/health/healthy_aging/healthy_connections/forgiveness-your-health-depends-on-it
3. https://www.mayoclinic.org/healthy-lifestyle/adult-health/in-depth/forgiveness/art-20047692

Too Blessed to be Stressed!
1. https://www.mayoclinic.org/healthy-lifestyle/stress-management/in-depth/stress/art-20046037

ADDiTiONAL RESOURCES

EPA Distributed Structure-Searchable Toxicity (DSSTox) Database is a listing chemical substances and supporting documentation.
- https://www.epa.gov/chemical-research/distributed-structure-searchable-toxicity-dsstox-database

CDC RESOURCES for Toxic Chemicals and Exposure
- https://www.cdc.gov/exposurereport/pdf/FourthReport_ExecutiveSummary.pdf
- https://www.cdc.gov/biomonitoring/chemical_factsheets.html
- https://www.cdc.gov/exposurereport/pdf/FourthReport_UpdatedTables_Volume1_Mar2018.pdf
- https://www.cdc.gov/exposurereport/pdf/FourthReport_UpdatedTables_Volume2_Mar2018.pdf
- https://www.cdc.gov/exposurereport/suggested_citations.html
- https://www.cdc.gov/exposurereport/faq.html
- https://www.cdc.gov/exposurereport/data_sources_analysis.html
- https://www.atsdr.cdc.gov/pfas/docs/pfas_fact_sheet.pdf
- https://www.atsdr.cdc.gov/docs/17_278160-A_PFAS-FamilyTree-508.pdf

- https://www.atsdr.cdc.gov/pfas/pfas-exposure.html
- https://www.atsdr.cdc.gov/pfas/health-effects.html
- https://www.niehs.nih.gov/health/materials/perflourinated_chemicals_508.pdf
- http://www.c8sciencepanel.org
- https://www.atsdr.cdc.gov/toxfaqs/tf.asp?id=1116&tid=237
- https://www.atsdr.cdc.gov/toxfaqs/tf.asp?id=1116&tid=237
- https://www.atsdr.cdc.gov/toxprofiles/tp.asp?id=1117&tid=237
- https://www.atsdr.cdc.gov/pfas/atsdr_sites_involvement.html
- https://www.cdc.gov/cdc-info

More on EMFs
- http://emwatch.com/emf-radiation-from-domestic-appliances/
- https://ehtrust.org/key-issues/the-environment-and-health/wireless-radiationelectromagnetic-fields-increases-toxic-body-burden/

Obesity and Metabolic Syndrome
- https://youtu.be/dBnniua6-oM Sugar: The Bitter Truth
- https://youtu.be/ceFyF9px20Y Fat Chance: Fructose 2.0

To contact Devra Betts, please visit her online:
Facebook: www.facebook.com/choosehealthforlife
Instagram: www.Instagram.com/devrabetts
Website: www.devrabetts.com
Email: devra@devrabetts.com

Made in the USA
San Bernardino, CA
16 February 2019